Boards Boot Camp

Step 1 USMLE & Level 1 COMLEX Preparation

Hi-Yield Compendium

Volume 2

Eleventh Edition

2014

Boards Boot Camp
Hi-Yield Compendium

11th Edition

Copyright 2014, Mindworks Corporation

Pro-Medica Publishing Company

ISBN 978-1-304-41229-4

Library of Congress Cataloging-in-Publication Data
Boards Boot Camp Hi-Yield Compendium – VOLUME 2/Lori A. Dolinski, MSc, PhD, DO – 11th ed.
ISBN 978-1-304-41229-4
1. Boards Boot Camp Hi-Yield Compendium   2. Dolinski, Lori A.

BOARDS BOOT CAMP HI-YIELD COMPENDIUM

Written by Lori A. Dolinski, MSc, PhD, DO
Illustrations by Karen S. High and Lori A. Dolinski, MSc, PhD, DO
Edited by Boards Boot Camp, Mindworks Corporation
Printed in the United States of America
Printed and Distributed by Lulu, Inc.
Published by Pro-Medica Publishing Company, PO Box 310, Revere, PA 18953.

PATHOLOGY

Bones and Joints

Skeletal Muscle Disorders

Neurology

Endocrinology

Dermatology

Toxicology

MICROBIOLOGY

Virology

Mycology

BIOCHEMISTRY

Cyclic AMP

Lipids

PHYSIOLOGY

ANATOMY

Embryology and Fetal Studies

High-Yield Anatomy Facts

PHARMACOLOGY

APPENDICES

A Note to the Student:

The Boards Boot Camp Hi-Yield Compendium for Step 1 USMLE and Level 1 COMLEX preparation is a hi-yield but extremely comprehensive collection of information that covers hundreds of must-know facts and concepts. It is an excellent stand-alone study guide and is also the cornerstone review text for all Boards Boot Camp Level 1 prep programs. You will find that concepts are presented in an easy-to-learn format that integrates conceptual understanding, key terms, linkage of related topics, and repetition through varying presentations to ensure that your boards preparation is thorough, accurate, up-to-date and successful.

Good luck and have fun!

PRO-MEDICA PUBLISHING COMPANY

VOLUME TWO

Section 54.0 BIOCHEMISTRY

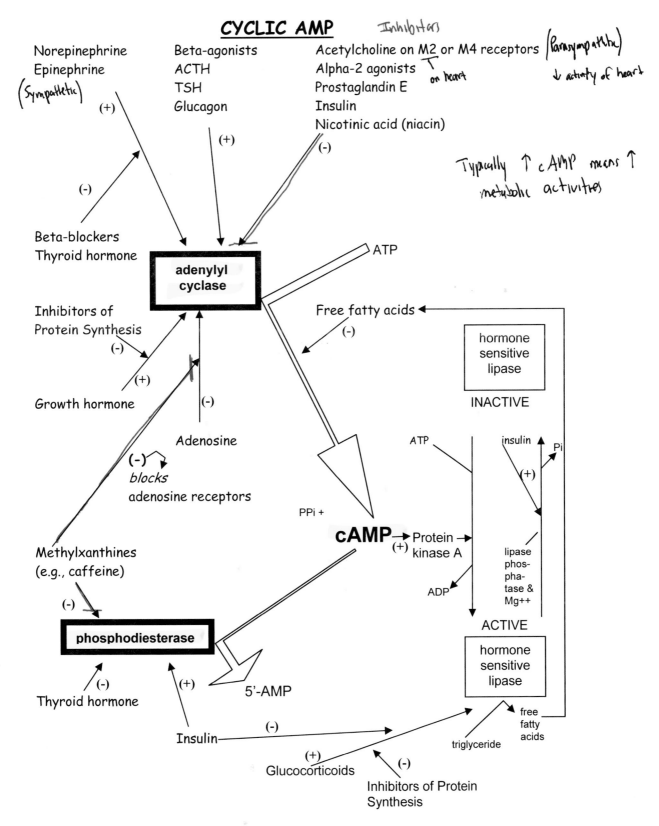

CYCLIC AMP

Inhibitors

| Norepinephrine Epinephrine (Sympathetic) | Beta-agonists ACTH TSH Glucagon | Acetylcholine on M2 or M4 receptors (Parasympathetic) Alpha-2 agonists — on heart ↓ activity of heart Prostaglandin E Insulin Nicotinic acid (niacin) |

(+) (+) (-)

Typically ↑ cAMP means ↑ metabolic activities

Beta-blockers
Thyroid hormone

(-)

adenylyl cyclase

ATP

Free fatty acids
(-)

hormone sensitive lipase
INACTIVE

Inhibitors of Protein Synthesis
(-)
(+)

Growth hormone

(-)

Adenosine

(-) ↘ *blocks* adenosine receptors

ATP

insulin Pi
(+)

PPi +

cAMP → Protein → kinase A
(+)

lipase phos-pha-tase & Mg++

ADP

ACTIVE

Methylxanthines (e.g., caffeine)

(-)

phosphodiesterase

hormone sensitive lipase

(-) (+)

5'-AMP

Thyroid hormone

free fatty acids

Insulin
(-)

triglyceride

(+)

Glucocorticoids (-)

Inhibitors of Protein Synthesis

Boards Boot Camp High-Yield Compendium

Section 55.0   LIPID METABOLISM

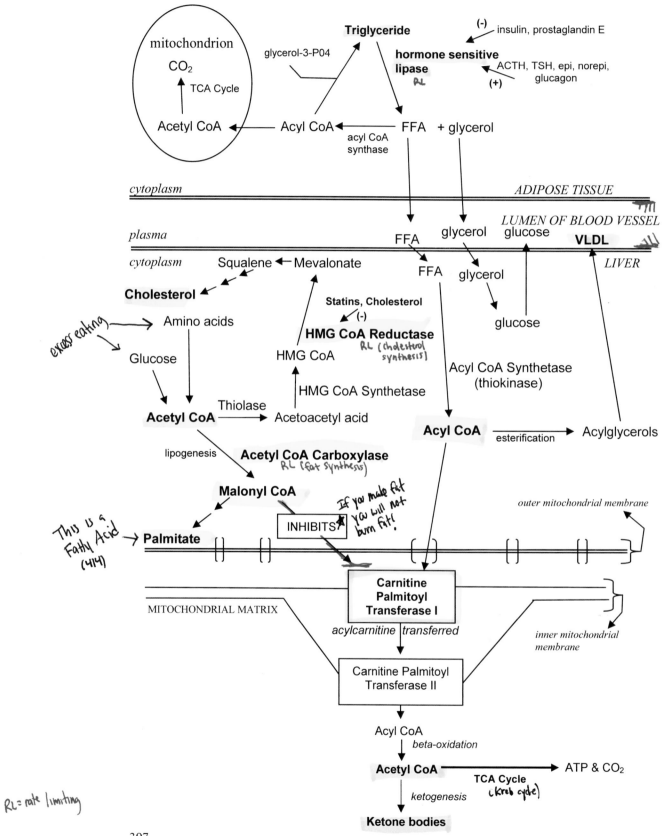

Boards Boot Camp High-Yield Compendium

Section 55.1   FATTY ACID SYNTHESIS

- **Acetyl CoA** is the substrate and palmitate is the end product
- Fatty acid synthesis occurs in many tissues: liver, kidney, brain, lung, mammary gland, and adipose tissue
- Acetyl CoA in the cell **CYTOPLASM**, when present in excess, will be metabolized to malonyl CoA
- **Malonyl CoA** production is catalyzed by the rate controlling enzyme for fat synthesis, **acetyl CoA carboxylase**
- Acetyl CoA carboxylase is stimulated by insulin and inhibited by glucagon and epinephrine
- Malonyl CoA will inhibit fatty acid metabolism by inhibiting carnitine palmitoyl transferase I, the enzyme responsible for ensuring entry of fatty acid-derived acyl CoA into the mitochondrion for metabolism
- Malonyl CoA undergoes several reactions that are catalyzed by **fatty acid synthase**
- Fatty acid synthase, a multienzyme complex, catalyzes the connection of one acetyl CoA molecule (a 2-carbon molecule) to 7 malonyl CoA molecules, causing the fatty acid chain to grow by 2 carbons for each malonyl CoA added; the final product is **palmitate** (a 16 carbon saturated fatty acid)
- Palmitate is a fatty acid, and is the sole fatty acid from which all other fatty acids are manufactured
- Other fatty acids are produced by malonyl CoA addition to the chain and/or catalysis by **fatty acyl-CoA desaturase**, an enzyme that introduces double bonds into fatty acids (thereby making them "unsaturated")

If you are synthesizing fat you will inhibit fat metabolism

Notes:

Boards Boot Camp High-Yield Compendium

Section 55.2   Clinical Issues: Fatty Acid Synthesis

- Those with **diabetes mellitus type I** are not able to manufacture insulin; even treated individuals occasionally have moments of insufficient insulin availability (available through administration). Lack of insulin results in decreased <u>acetyl CoA carboxylase</u> activity. Without this enzyme, less fatty acids and, therefore, fewer triglycerides are made. This accounts, in part, for the **thin body habitus** most with Type I diabetes have.

  low insulin
  ↓
  less lipid synthesis

- Overeating causes abundant insulin release in the ordinary patient. The food provides plentiful substrate for acetyl CoA manufacture by ensuring a ready supply of glucose and amino acids. The insulin stimulates acetyl CoA carboxylase activity, too, spurring on fatty acid synthesis. The result is excess triglyceride synthesis and **obesity**.

- **Lipogenesis is strongly encouraged by ingestion of sucrose (table sugar; comprised of <u>fructose</u> + glucose) and <u>fructose</u> (high fructose corn syrup** used as a sweetener in numerous processed foods) since the fructose does not undergo the first rate-controlling steps of glycolysis, and instead enters glycolysis late in the process; this makes its metabolite quickly and suddenly flood the cytoplasm, eventually providing a generous supply of acetyl CoA for fatty acid synthesis.

- **Essential fatty acids** are fatty acids essential to our diet since we cannot manufacture them; they include linolenic acid and linoleic acid.

- **Trans-fatty acids** are found in partially hydrogenated vegetable oils (e.g., margarine). They are metabolized like saturated fatty acids.

Section 55.3   KETOGENESIS

- Occurs exclusively in the **liver mitochondria**
- Occurs mostly in the context of **Type I diabetes mellitus and starvation**
- Any **very high rate of fatty acid oxidation** (triglyceride metabolism with fatty acid break-down) will result in ketogenesis (the production of ketone bodies)
- Type I diabetics who do not have adequate insulin administration have a deficiency in insulin; insulin normally inhibits the enzyme that initiates and acts as the rate-limiter to triglyceride metabolism, hormone sensitive lipase. Hence, triglyceride metabolism occurs faster than usual. However, that alone rarely causes clinically significant ketogenesis. An ADDITIONAL activation of hormone sensitive lipase is necessary. A potent activator is epinephrine (adrenalin). So, the combination of lack of insulin (such as can only be experienced by a Type I diabetic) + a physically or emotionally disruptive event that causes epinephrine release will allow for EXCESSIVE hormone sensitive lipase activity, resulting in EXCESSIVE triglyceride

401

metabolism and fatty acid oxidation. The result is that the TCA cycle is saturated with acetyl CoA, allowing the excess acetyl CoA to be metabolized to ketone bodies. This results in DKA (diabetic ketoacidosis)

- Persons who are starving will have extremely low insulin levels + high epinephrine, allowing for ketone body synthesis secondary to excessive triglyceride metabolism. A mild ketosis occurs.

- The **ketone bodies are acids ("ketoacids")** and include **acetoacetate, 3-hydroxybutyrate, and acetone** (the latter smells fruity on the breath of those with ketoacidosis)

Section 55.4   Clinical Issues: Ketogenesis

- **Type I diabetes mellitus** (without insulin and with increased epinephrine release) or **starvation** promote increased triglyceride metabolism and, therefore, increased fatty acid oxidation. The result is excess acetyl CoA and the metabolism of the excess to ketone bodies.

- **Carnitine deficiency** can be seen in the premature infant (due to inadequate biosynthesis) or in the hemodialysis patient (due to dialysis-related losses)
  - ➢ As a result, carnitine palmitoyl transferases levels are low.
  - ➢ This leads to decreased fatty acid oxidation
  - ➢ Ketone bodies are never made
  - ➢ There is raised plasma FFA (free fatty acids) because they are not metabolized appropriately

➤ The plasma FFAs cause hypoglycemia due to decreased gluconeogenesis

➤ The same signs occur in **Reye's Syndrome** (although carnitine levels are normal in Reye's – the exact molecular cause is unknown)

Boards Boot Camp High-Yield Compendium

Section 55.5   EICOSANOIDS

- These are a type of unsaturated fatty acid

- They are all derived from eicosanoic fatty acids which, themselves, are derived exclusively from essential *(need & dont make)* fatty acids ("EFAs;" linolenic and linoleic acids) *make all others from Palmitate*

- The major eicosanoid is arachidonic acid.

- Arachidonic acid is present in all cell membranes (as part of many of the phospholipids that make up the phospholipid bilayer)

- Arachidonic acid is the precursor to prostaglandins, thromboxane, and leukotrienes.

- *Steroid* ⊥ Phospholipase A2 catalyzes the removal of arachidonic acid from membrane phospholipids, and cyclooxygenase ├ *NSAID Aspirin* catalyzes the metabolism of arachidonic acid to prostaglandins (and, later, thromboxane); lipoxygenase catalyzes the metabolism of arachidonic acid to leukotrienes.
  - ➢ Prostaglandins cause vasodilation, exudation, and pain
  - ➢ Thromboxanes cause platelet aggregation and vasoconstriction
  - ➢ Leukotrienes cause POTENT bronchoconstriction

Section 55.6   <u>FATTY ACIDS</u>

How to read notation:

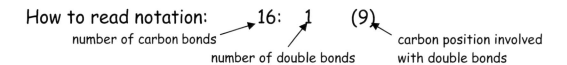

number of carbon bonds → 16: 1 (9)

number of double bonds

carbon position involved with double bonds

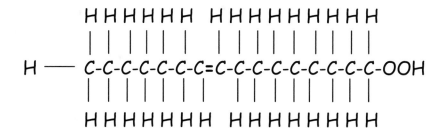

Fatty Acid Terminology:

Numbering (#) Method   #1 carbon = <u>C</u> OOH

Greek Method   etc – C – C – COOH
                              β   α

Greek ω (omega)
                              last carbon
                              C – C – C---------------COOH
                              ω_1 ω_2 ω_3

MONO-UNSATURATED: (have one C=C double bond)
Palmitoleic acid   16:1(9)
Oleic acid   18:1(9)

POLY-UNSATURATED: (have several C=C double bonds)
Linoleic acid   18:2(9,12)
Linolenic acid   18:3(9,12,15)
Arachidonic acid   20:4(5,8,11,14)

SATURATED: (have no C=C double bonds)
Precursor → Palmitic acid   16:0
Stearic acid   18:0

Boards Boot Camp High-Yield Compendium

Section 55.7   **CHOLESTEROL SYNTHESIS**

❖ Synthesis occurs in cells throughout the body
❖ The substrate is acetyl CoA and the end-product is cholesterol.
❖ The rate-limiting step of cholesterol synthesis is controlled by HMG-CoA reductase.
❖ HMG-CoA reductase is the site of action of the drugs known as HMG-CoA reductase inhibitors (statins)
❖ HMG-CoA reductase is activated by insulin and inhibited by glucagon, glucocorticoids, and cholesterol
❖ Because of insulin's effect on HMG CoA reductase, ingestion of a glucose- or amino-acid rich meal will promote cholesterol synthesis; furthermore, the excess glucose and amino acids will serve as substrate to cholesterol synthesis. This is why a diet free of overeating is as important as a low cholesterol diet in limiting serum cholesterol levels.

Section 55.7.1   **CHOLESTEROL FUNCTIONS**

Cholesterol is:
1) necessary for all human cell plasma membranes, and is an integral component as an embedded molecule within the phospholipid bilayer
2) the precursor for all other steroids in the body, such as corticosteroids (cortisol), mineralocorticoids (aldosterone), sex hormones (estrogen, progesterone, testosterone), bile acids, and vitamin D
3) is derived from the diet + endogenous manufacture in the body
4) is abundant in egg yolk, meat, liver, and CNS tissues

Section 55.8   <u>BILE ACIDS</u>

The ring structure of cholesterol (the "sterol ring") cannot be fully metabolized by humans; therefore, the ring must be eliminated by:

   (1) conversion to bile acids which are excreted to feces
                      <u>OR</u>
   (2) secretion of cholesterol (intact) into bile which is eliminated to feces

Bile acids act as emulsifiers in the intestine, allowing for better absorption of lipids. Bile acids and intact cholesterol are carried through the bile ducts to the intestine via bile.

2 Types of Bile Acids:
   1. Primary – made in liver from cholesterol
   2. Secondary – made in intestine from bile acids; done by bacteria

If the bile acids are conjugated to glycine and taurine (most are; this is done in liver), they become bile salts.

Only about 3.5% of all bile salts and bile acids in intestine are ultimately excreted with feces; all the remainder is reabsorbed in the ileum and taken back to the liver via the portal system (and carried on albumin).

Boards Boot Camp High-Yield Compendium

Section 55.9   **Clinical Issues: Disorders due to Excess Cholesterol**

❖ **Atherosclerosis** – which may lead to MI, CVA, PVD (peripheral vascular disease), mesenteric ischemia, and aortic aneurysm; atherosclerosis is initiated by the deposition of excess LDL-cholesterol in serum onto intima (inner lining of blood vessels) which, then, leads to an inflammatory reaction with macrophages.

[handwritten: make lipoprotein lipase = start gravy w/ TG]
[handwritten: foam cells, platelets next / IL1 TNF]

❖ **Gallstones** (cholelithiasis) – which can predispose one to cholecystitis, choledocholithiasis, and ascending cholangitis; excess cholesterol in bile precipitates out to form stones

[handwritten: cholesterol ↓ liver ↓ or ↘ Bile / VLDL]

❖ **Xanthomas** – the accumulation of cholesterol-laden macrophages in various body structures, including tendons, skin, and other locations.

Section 55.10   **LIPID STRUCTURES**

TRIGLYCERIDES

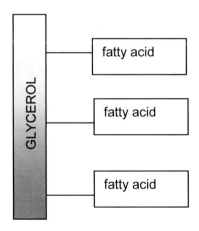

GLYCEROPHOSPHOLIPIDS

The glycerol-phospholipids are what we generically term "phospholipids," and are the components to the lipid bilayer.

All membranes are comprised of a "phospholipid bilayer" – two layers of phospholipids.

There are many types of phospholipids:
Phosphatidyl choline⟶the primary component of surfactant
Phosphatidyl ethanolamine⟶the 2 most abundant phospholipids
                                     in human eukaryotes
Phosphatidyl serine
Phosphatidyl inositol
Cardiolipin → the only one that is antigenic to humans

Syphilis
SLE

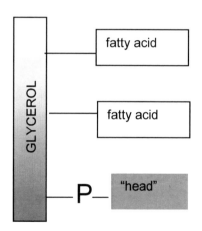

Note that all phospholipids have 2 fatty acids. Different types of fatty acids can make up the phospholipid; hence, all cell membranes are comprised of phospholipids with a variety of fatty acids and heads attached. Some of those membrane phospholipids contain a fatty acid known as arachidonic acid. When those phospholipids are liberated from the membrane, phospholipase A2 can remove the arachidonic acid for future metabolism to prostaglandins, thromboxanes, and leukotrienes.

GLYCOLIPIDS = ceramide + sugar(s)

A special type of glycolipid is the ganglioside:
   GANGLIOSIDE = ceramide + oligosaccharide + NANA
            (NANA = N-acetylneuraminic acid)

Another type of glycolipid is the cerebroside

Ceramide (a component of glycolipid)

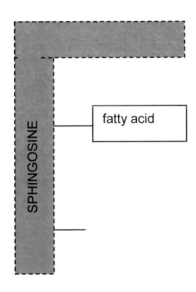

Sphingosine (a component of ceramide)

Boards Boot Camp High-Yield Compendium

Cerebroside (a type of glycolipid; note it is ceramide + sugar)

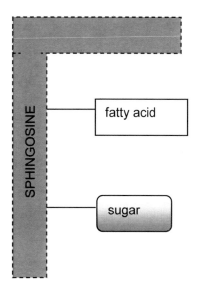

Ganglioside (a type of glycolipid; note it contains ceramide + sugars)

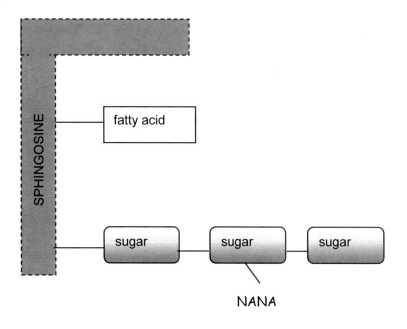

Boards Boot Camp High-Yield Compendium

SPHINGOLIPIDS

Sphingolipids are also known as sphingophospholipids. They
make up, along with long chain FAs, the bulk of the myelin sheath that
insulates nerve fibers of the CNS (sphingomyelin is the primary
sphingolipid that plays this role) → this is why
sphingolipidoses are <u>SO</u> destructive to CNS

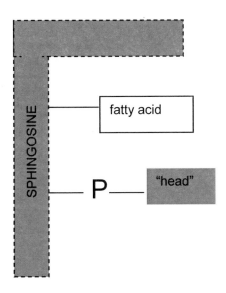

Sphingomyelin is a sphingolipid, and is particularly prevalent in the CNS. It is a sphingolipid because it is comprised of sphingosine + a fatty acid + a head (which, in this case, is choline)

Sphingomyelin = sphingosine + FA + choline

Ceramide

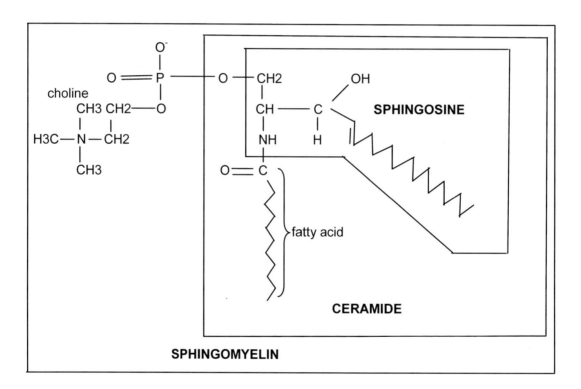

Boards Boot Camp High-Yield Compendium

SPHINGOLIPIDOSES

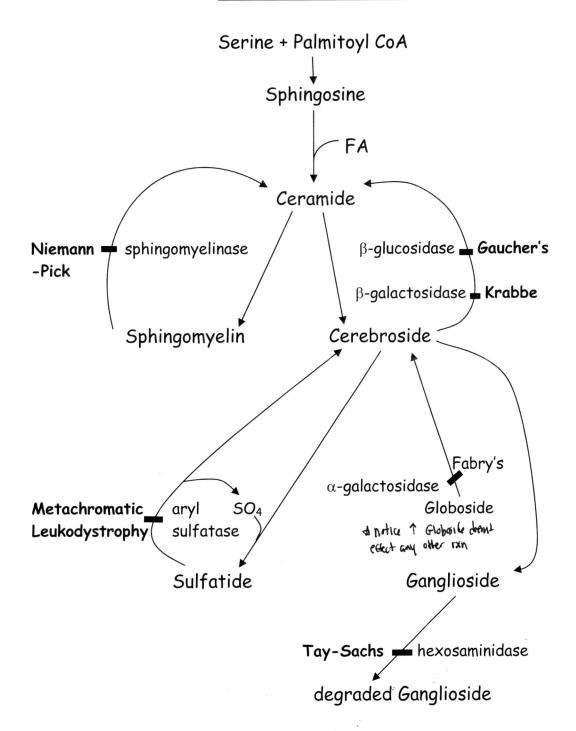

Sphingolipidoses are disorders marked by an inability to metabolize or degrade certain sphingolipids, resulting in the accumulation of certain sphingolipids. It is a result of dysfunction of cellular lysosomes. All sphingolipidoses, except Fabry's Disease, result in serious CNS disorders. (AR)   (XR)

(1) **NIEMANN-PICK** ⋆ hepatomegaly, splenomegaly
MR/ID (intellectual disability) –
  severe!!
Fatal in early life
Cherry red macula

(2) **GAUCHER'S** hepatomegaly, splenomegaly
MR/ID
Erosion of long bones/osteoporosis

Ashkenazi Jews

(3) **KRABBE'S** MR/ID (severe!!!)
Blindness, deafness, convulsions,
  paralysis (due to *almost*
  complete absence of myelin)
Fatal in early life

(4) **FABRY'S** Angiokeratomas
Reddish-purple rash
Kidney failure
Heart failure

(5) **METACHROMATIC** MR/ID
  DYSTROPHY Psychiatric problems, dementia
Progressive paralysis

(6) **TAY-SACHS** MR/ID
Cherry red macula, blindness
⋆ none

Ashkenazi Jews

Section 56.0   DIGESTIVE ENZYMES

1)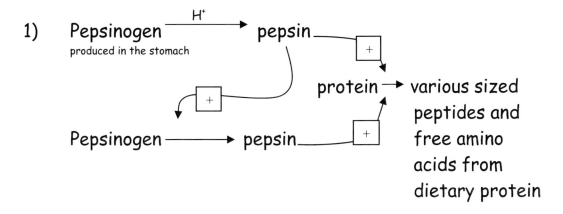

2)   Enteropeptidase – produced by the duodenal mucosa
                  - randomly cleaves dietary proteins +
                  converts trypsinogen to trypsin

3)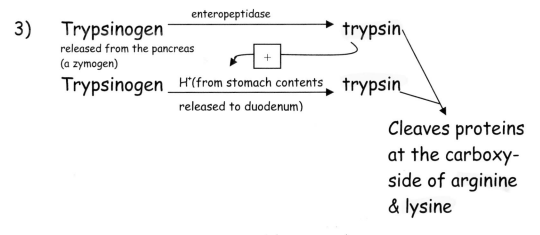

     Cleaves proteins
     at the carboxy-
     side of arginine
     & lysine

4)   Chymotrypsinogen ⟶ chymotrypsin ⟶ cleaves
       released by pancreas   trypsin   protein at
                                                 the carboxy-
                                                 side of
                                                 phenylalanine,
                                                 tyrosine,
                                                 tryptophan, or
                                                 leucine

5)   Proelastase ⟶ Elastase ⟶ cleaves elastin
       released by pancreas   trypsin

6) Procarboxypeptidase A $\xrightarrow{\text{trypsin}}$ carboxypeptidases
    Procarboxypeptidase B ⟋ A & B

                         Cleave proteins 1 amino acid at a time
                             from the carboxy-end

7) Lactase $\longrightarrow$ cleaves lactose into galactose & glucose
    produced by brush border

The peptide products of the enzymatic cleavages are absorbed
by the brush border of the intestine.

Section 57.0   <u>AMINO ACIDS – METABOLISM</u>

PHENYLALANINE

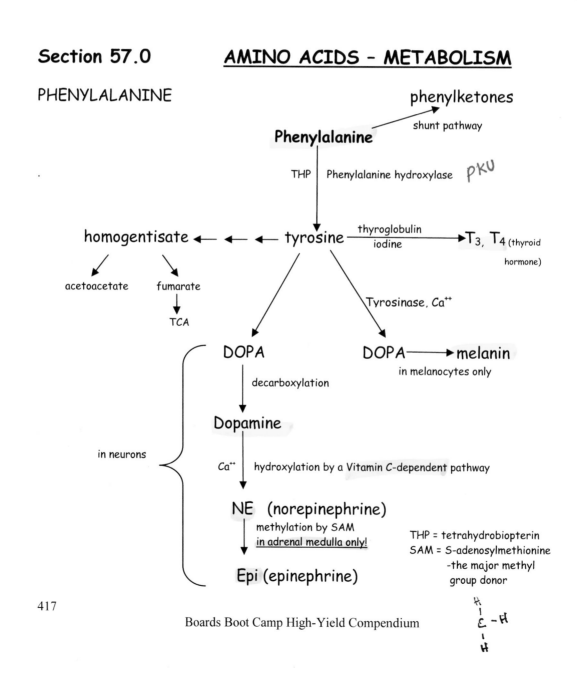

THP = tetrahydrobiopterin
SAM = S-adenosylmethionine
-the major methyl group donor

Boards Boot Camp High-Yield Compendium

TRYPTOPHAN

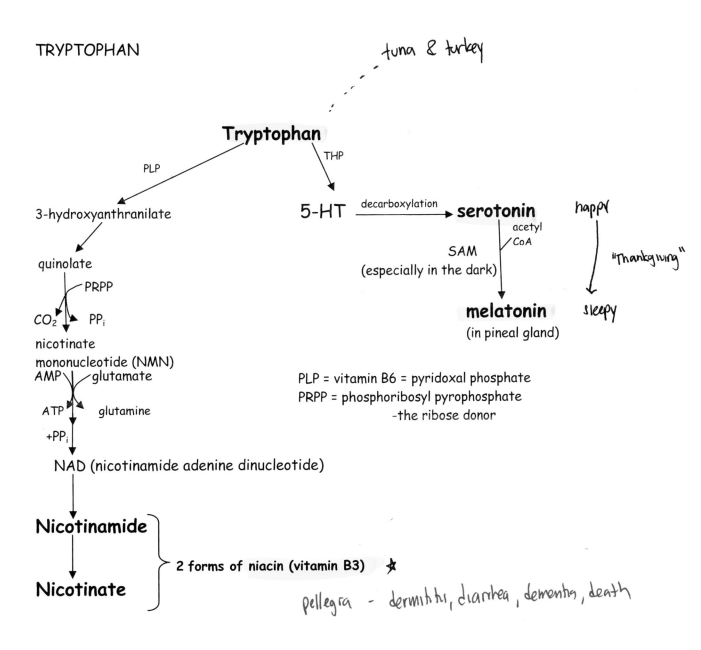

tuna & turkey

Tryptophan

PLP → 3-hydroxyanthranilate

THP → 5-HT — decarboxylation → **serotonin**   happy

quinolate

PRPP

CO_2 ↓ ↗ PP_i

nicotinate
mononucleotide (NMN)

AMP ↘ ↙ glutamate

ATP ↓ ↗ glutamine

+PP_i

NAD (nicotinamide adenine dinucleotide)

Nicotinamide

Nicotinate

} 2 forms of niacin (vitamin B3) ☆

SAM
(especially in the dark)

acetyl
CoA

melatonin
(in pineal gland)

"Thanksgiving"

sleepy

PLP = vitamin B6 = pyridoxal phosphate
PRPP = phosphoribosyl pyrophosphate
-the ribose donor

pellegra - dermihihi, diarrhea, dementia, death

In serotonin (carcinoid) syndrome most tryptophan is
used to make 5-HT instead of niacin
so you get a niacin def.

GLUTAMATE & GABA

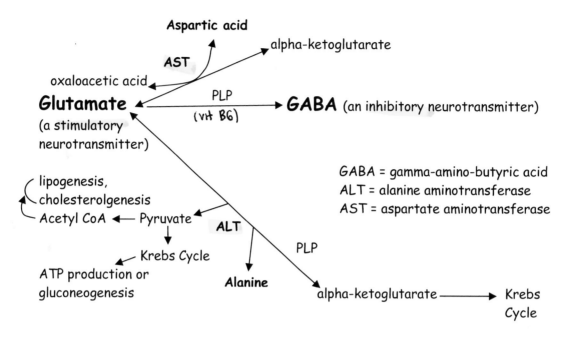

GABA = gamma-amino-butyric acid
ALT = alanine aminotransferase
AST = aspartate aminotransferase

Glycine is amino acid making heme

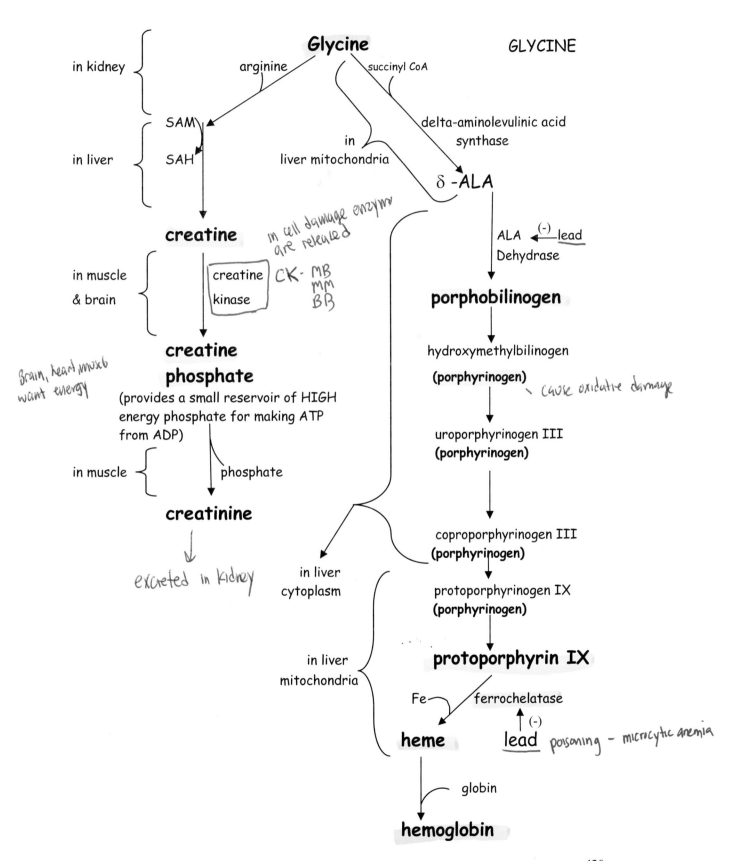

Glycine

GLYCINE

in kidney
arginine
succinyl CoA

SAM
in
liver mitochondria
delta-aminolevulinic acid
synthase

in liver
SAH
δ-ALA

creatine
ALA (-) lead
Dehydrase

in cell damage enzymes are released

in muscle & brain
creatine kinase
CK- MB MM BB

porphobilinogen

creatine phosphate

hydroxymethylbilinogen
(porphyrinogen)
cause oxidative damage

Brain, heart, musc6 want energy

(provides a small reservoir of HIGH energy phosphate for making ATP from ADP)

uroporphyrinogen III
(porphyrinogen)

in muscle
phosphate

coproporphyrinogen III
(porphyrinogen)

creatinine

in liver cytoplasm

protoporphyrinogen IX
(porphyrinogen)

excreted in kidney

in liver mitochondria

protoporphyrin IX

Fe
ferrochelatase

heme
lead (-) poisoning - microcytic anemia

globin

hemoglobin

420

Boards Boot Camp High-Yield Compendium

HISTIDINE

Histidine $\xrightarrow{\text{PLP}}$ **Histamine** $\longrightarrow$ exudation, bronchoconstriction, HCl secretion
in stomach

ARGININE
Arginine $\xrightarrow{\text{NADPH}}$ citrulline + NO + NADP
$\downarrow$
vasodilation

Section 57.1   Methylation of Molecules

S-adenosyl methionine cycle: How Molecules are Methylated

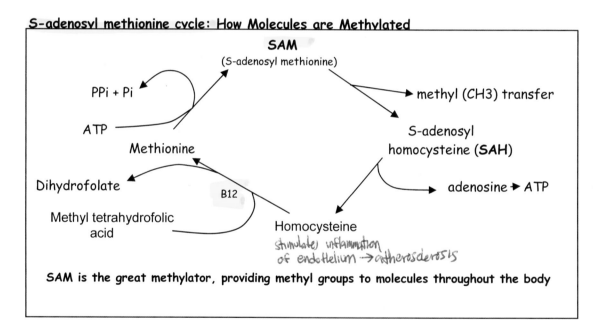

SAM is the great methylator, providing methyl groups to molecules throughout the body

B12 can ↓ homocysteine to ↓ inflammation

Section 57.2   **Enzyme Disorders**

Disease	Defect	Result	S&S
Albinism	tyrosinase deficiency X-Linked = ocular albinism AR = oculocutaneous dbinism	no melanin made	1) unpigmented eyes +/- hair and skin 2) increased squamous cell CA, melanoma, — melanocyte present actinic keratosis
Phenylketonuria (PKU)	phenylalanine hydroxylase deficiency OR defect in THP production	phenyl ketones accumulate & decreased DOPA, Epi, NE produced	1) musty odor of urine ketones 2) hypopigmentation 3) intellectual disability (MR/ID) phenyl ketones are neuro toxic Tx = Phe-free diet
Alkaptonuria	homogentisate oxidase deficiency	homogentisate increases, then auto-oxidizes; these oxidants poly-merize to form dark pigments (brownish black)	1) degenerative arthritis 2) darkly pigmented urine (when exposed to air) 3) pigmentation of connective tissue (ochronosis)

Boards Boot Camp High-Yield Compendium

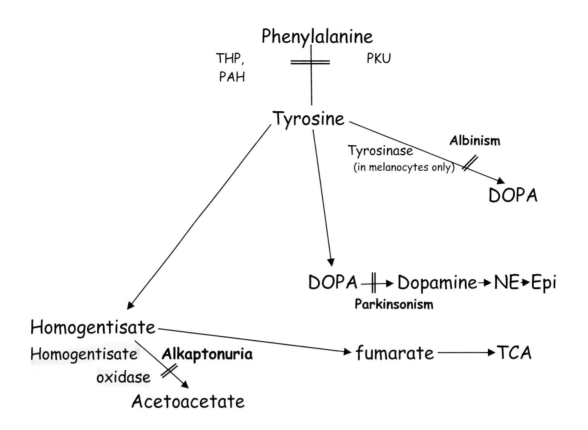

Phenylalanine

THP,
PAH | PKU

Tyrosine

Tyrosinase
(in melanocytes only) — Albinism → DOPA

Tyrosine → Homogentisate

Tyrosine → DOPA → Dopamine → NE → Epi

Parkinsonism

Homogentisate → fumarate → TCA

Homogentisate
oxidase — Alkaptonuria → Acetoacetate

Maple Syrup Urine

Disease   α-ketoacid   accumulation of   1) urine smells like
  -AR   dehydrogenase   branched chain   maple syrup or
         deficiency   amino acids   burnt sugar
                     (isoleucine, leucine,   2) evident by week
                     valine)   1 of age; extensive
                                         brain damage
                                         occurs

Tx = PRIOR to 1 week of age;   concomitantly
       dietary proteins <u>free</u>   ↓
       of BCAA   **MR/ID!!**

Dx = enzyme assay at birth

                 Highest incidence <u>in world</u> is in
                 Old Order Mennonites of
                 Lancaster & Lebanon Counties,
                 PA

Homocystinuria cystathionine homocysteine 1) **MR/ID**
synthase accumulates, 2) lens dislocation
deficiency then is 3) increased CAD
auto- 4) traps adenosine as
oxidized SAH: without free
homocystine adenosine for body, a
limited amount of ATP
is made
Dx = enzyme assay → decreased
Tx = decreased methionine diet and cognition (MR/ID)
HIGH B6 supplementation 5) the increased
to maximize any even partly homocysteine causes
functional cystathionine increased platelet
synthase, aggregation &
+ B12 and folate supplements endothelial
to shunt off accumulated damage (therefore,
homocysteine increased CAD and
CVA risk)

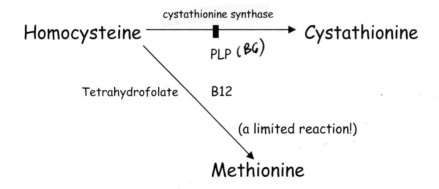

cystathionine synthase

Homocysteine ———————■————→ Cystathionine

PLP (B6)

Tetrahydrofolate   B12

(a limited reaction!)

Methionine

Cystinuria   defect in   in the kidney and   1) cystine urolithiasis
                              membrane   and collecting
                              transport   system, the high cysteine is
                              of dibasic   oxidized to cystine, resulting
                              amino acids   in urolithiasis
                              (cysteine,
                              ornithine,
COAL   arginine,   *Peed at → black stones*
                              and lysine),
                              impairing
                              renal
                              reabsorption
                              of these
                              amino acids

Hartnup Disease

defect in   decreased serum   1) yields niacin deficiency:
membrane   tryptophan   pellagra
transport
of tryptophan,
impairing
renal
reabsorption
and
impairing
intestinal
uptake of tryptophan

Boards Boot Camp High-Yield Compendium

Section 57.2.1   Enzyme Characteristics and Kinetics

- **Enzymes** catalyze reactions.

- Most enzymes are **proteins**.

- Enzymes convert substrate into product; the **substrate binds to the enzyme at the active site** and, via enzymatic action, is converted into a product molecule.

- Enzymes are typically very selective for a particular substrate, and carry out very specific reactions.

- Enzymes work in several different ways, each of which work to **lower the Gibbs energy**; in other words, they lower the energy needed to bring about a reaction whereby substrate becomes product.

- **Some enzymes are subject to allosteric modulation**; this means that they have allosteric sites (besides the active site) on them that bind molecules in the cell's environment. These molecules form weak, non-covalent bonds with these allosteric sites, but, in so doing, cause a change in conformation of the enzyme. The change in conformation also affects the active site, thus affecting the rate of reaction.

- **Cofactors** are inorganic molecules that bind at areas OTHER than the active site to augment enzymatic activity. Examples of cofactors are minerals like iron, selenium, etc.

- **Coenzymes** are organic molecules that bind at areas OTHER than the active site to augment enzymatic activity. Examples of coenzymes are vitamins.

- Enzymes that require cofactors or coenzymes, but have none bound, are called **apoenzymes**. Those with cofactors or coenzymes bound are called **holoenzymes**.

- **Enzyme kinetics** refers to how enzymes bind to substrates and catalyze their conversion to products. Most enzymes can catalyze several MILLION reactions per second!

- **Enzyme rate** (the rate it can carry out a reaction) is dependent upon substrate concentration, plus, generally, temperature, pH, and salt concentration.

- The maximum *rate* at which an enzyme can produce product is **Vmax**.

- However, substrate concentration as it relates to and affects enzyme activity is expressed through the **Michaelis-Menten constant (Km)**.

- **Km** = ½ **Vmax** = the substrate concentration required for an enzyme to reach one-half of its maximum reaction rate.

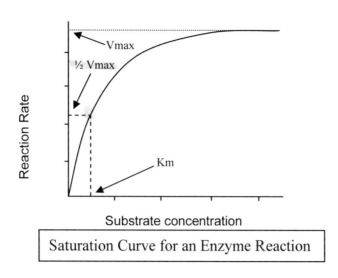

Saturation Curve for an Enzyme Reaction

$\uparrow$ km = $\downarrow$ affinity
$\downarrow$ km = $\uparrow$ affinity

- **The higher the Km** for any particular substrate, the more substrate is necessary to help the enzyme achieve half of its maximal speed of catalyzing reactions.

- The higher the Km, the **lower the affinity of substrate for enzyme** (e.g., the substrate has not very likely to bind the enzyme)

- **The lower the Km** for any particular substrate, the less substrate is necessary to help the enzyme achieve half of its maximal speed to catalyzing reactions.

- The lower the Km for any particular substrate, the **higher the affinity of substrate for enzyme** (e.g., substrate is extremely likely to bind well to enzyme).

- Enzymatic reactions can be inhibited by various types of **enzyme inhibitors.**

- <u>There are 4 types of enzyme inhibitors:</u>

  Competitive inhibitors
  Uncompetitive inhibitors
  Non-competitive inhibitors
  Mixed inhibitors

- **Competitive inhibitors** bind to the active site (where substrate normally binds), thus competing with substrate for that active site.
  - The higher the competitive inhibitor concentration, the less substrate can bind, and the less enzymatic activity occurs.
  - Vmax is not changed, but Km is ~~reduced?~~ *increased* (meaning that more substrate is necessary for enzyme to even reach half of its maximal rate).
  - Example: disulfiram (Antabuse) on aldehyde oxidase

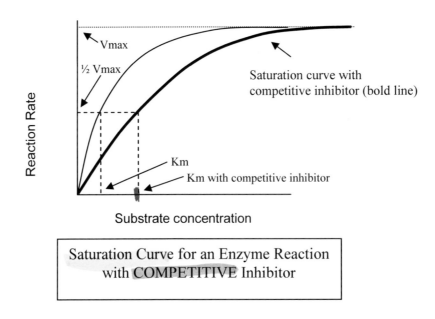

Saturation Curve for an Enzyme Reaction
with COMPETITIVE Inhibitor

Boards Boot Camp High-Yield Compendium

- **Uncompetitive inhibitors** can ONLY bind to the enzyme WHILE the substrate is bound; uncompetitive inhibitors render the enzyme completely inactive.
    - This is the rarest form of inhibition.

- **Non-competitive inhibitors** bind to the enzyme at a location other than the active site, thus NOT competing with substrate binding. That is why these are "non-competitive."
    - This type of inhibition is NOT influenced by substrate concentration, since there is no competition.
    - Vmax is reduced, but Km remains the same.

Vmax with non-competitive inhibitor

Vmax

½ Vmax

Saturation curve with non-competitive inhibitor (bold line)

½ Vmax with non-competitive inhibitor

Km

Reaction Rate

Substrate concentration

Saturation Curve for an Enzyme Reaction with NON-COMPETITIVE Inhibitor

- **Mixed inhibitors** resemble non-competitive inhibitors in "where" they bind, but, unlike non-competitive inhibitors, still allow for residual enzymatic activity despite their inhibiting effects.
  - They do not follow Michaelis-Menten principles
  - Many negative feedback systems in the body rely in this form of inhibition

- All inhibitors are either **reversible or irreversible**.

- **Most are reversible** (e.g., inhibitor leaves the enzyme, thus reversing the inhibition effect).

- **Irreversible inhibitors** bind covalently (permanently) with the enzyme, thus having a never-ending effect of inhibition on the enzyme.
  - Examples include eflornithine (for African Sleeping Sickness), aspirin, penicillin, and organophosphates (pesticides and nerve agents)

Boards Boot Camp High-Yield Compendium

Section 58.0   <u>CARBOHYDRATES</u>

Hexoses = 6 carbon sugars

There are 2 configurations:

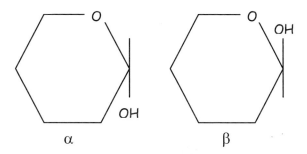

1) **digestible sugars are α (alpha)**
   EXCEPTION: lactose (galactose – beta 1,4 – glucose)
   Lactose is a beta sugar but, because of the enzyme known a lactase, we are able to digest it.

2) **indigestible sugars are β (beta)**
   Examples are chitin, pectin, and cellulose. Indigestible sugars are fiber. Soluble fibers can dissolve in water, and include pectin. Cellulose, the main plant fiber, is an insoluble fiber.

All 6-carbon sugars that enter the cell must first be phosphorylated (a phosphate group added to the molecule) before the sugar can be utilized in any metabolic pathway.

Hexo- & glucokinase → 6 carbon sugars require phosphorylation before they can be used; these are the enzymes that catalyze the phosphorylation

Boards Boot Camp High-Yield Compendium

	HEXOKINASE	**GLUCOKINASE**
Tissues	most	<u>liver</u>, β-islet cells
Substrate specificity	hexoses (with increased affinity for glucose)	glucose <u>only</u>
Affinity	high	low (therefore, only works when glucose is at VERY high concentrations)
V$_{max}$("capacity")	low	high "glucokinase is a glutton"
(-) feedback by G-6-P*	yes	no
Presence	constitutive (always available)	inducible
Function	ensure a supply of glucose for tissues, as well as avail other hexoses to cells	to remove glucose from blood following a meal

*G-6-P = glucose-6-phosphate

Monosaccharide = 1 sugar

Disaccharide = 2 sugars

Maltose	glucose + glucose	α1,4
Lactose	galactose + glucose	β1,4
Sucrose	glucose + fructose	α1,2

Polysaccharide = many sugars

Starch	glucoses only	α1.4 & α1.6
Glycogen	glucoses only	α1,4 & α1,6
Cellulose	glucoses only	β1,4
Chitin	glucoses, with amino groups	β1,4

Section 58.1   SACCHARIDE DISORDERS

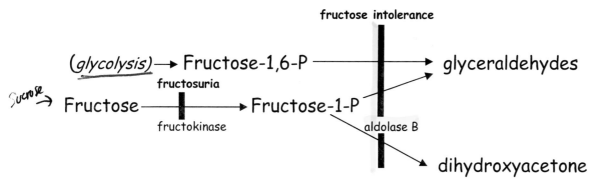

fructose intolerance

(*glycolysis*) → Fructose-1,6-P ————→ glyceraldehydes

Sucrose →

fructosuria

Fructose ——|——→ Fructose-1-P

fructokinase

aldolase B

→ dihydroxyacetone

Disease	Defect	Result	S&S, Comments
Fructosuria	fructokinase *now cant phosphorylate Fructose*	increased serum fructose	1. fructose is excreted in urine ("Fructosuria") 2. May lead to incorrect initial assumption of DM 3. autosomal recessive 4. Benign!
Fructose Intolerance	aldolase B	accumulation of fructose-1-PO$_4$ and fructose-1,6-PO$_4$	1. NOT benign!!! 2. Fructose-1-P builds up in kidney and liver, resulting in renal and liver failure

*Because aldolase B also operates in glycolysis, this disease causes accumulation of fructose-1,6-PO$_4$ and all other molecules before it **in glycolysis**, including:*

Glucose-6-PO$_4$

↓

glycogenolysis and gluconeogenesis are shut down due to G-6-P accumulation

↓

dangerous hypoglycemia, especially between meals

Disease	Defect	Result	S&S, Comments
Lactose Intolerance	lactase	increased lactose within intestinal lumen	1. lactose is a product of the mammary gland, and so is found in milk products 2. lactose intolerance occurs normally in 75% of adults of all ethnic groups except of NW European origin (almost 100% of US blacks have it by age 20) 3. flatus, bloating, borborygmi, diarrhea

β-hexose that is insoluble w/ lipase

Dx: 1) stool pH <6
2) lactose tolerance test (give 50g lactose, get symptoms in 20-30 min.; later, give 50g glucose and get no S&S but do get an increase in serum glucose) = (+) TEST)

Tx: lactose-free diet or lactase tablets with dairy ingestion

osmotic
↓
lose bowel

Bacteria use Lactose to make gas → flatus

Disease	Defect	Result	S&S, Comments
Galactosuria	galactose-1-PO$_4$ uridylyl transferase	accumulation of galactose-1-P &, therefore, also build-up of galactose	1. autosomal rec. 2. increased serum galactose 3. intracellular increase in galactose-1-P interferes with MANY metabolic processes → resulting in MR/ID and physical stunting. Also, galactose-1-P depletes liver of PO$_4$, resulting in liver failure (no ATP); the trapped PO$_4$ also exacerbates the MR/ID (intellectual disability).

*within a few weeks after birth and after being fed milk, infant becomes anorexic, vomits, stops growing, and becomes icteric.

*cataracts occur in fetus in utero if mother is galactosemic (and uncontrolled)

Dx = high serum galactose-1-PO$_4$
      low galactose -1-PO$_4$ uridylyl transferase

Tx = eliminate milk and milk products

→ even with tx, patients remain underachievers (even with normal IQ)

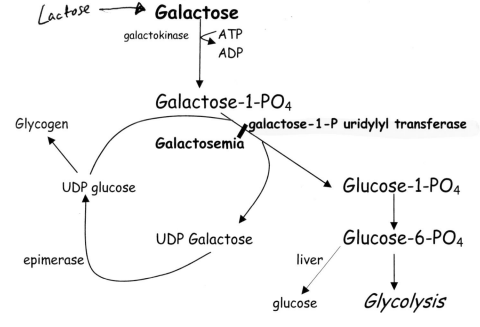

Section 59.0   GLYCOGEN STORAGE DISEASES

Normally, glucose is polymerized to form glycogen, a storage
form of glucose. Synthesis of glycogen occurs in kidney, muscle, & liver
(especially in the latter); so, the glycogen storage diseases have their
primary effect on liver and/or muscle.

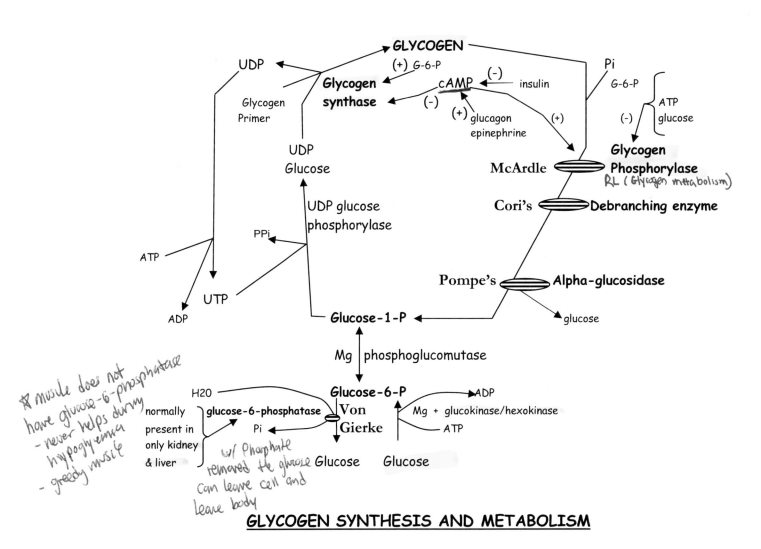

GLYCOGEN SYNTHESIS AND METABOLISM

Boards Boot Camp High-Yield Compendium

Glycogen Storage Diseases

Disease	Defect	Effect	S & S, Comments
Type I (Von Gierke)	lack of G-6-P phosphatase	accumulation of G-6-P &, so, also G-1-P	1. G-6-P is also the major product of gluconeogenesis; because of lack of G-6-phosphatase, it cannot become glucose via gluconeogenesis. Instead, the excess G-6P stimulates glycogenesis even if the patient is hypoglycemic! 2. G-1-P naturally inhibits glycogen phosphorylase. So, the increased G-1-P assures that glycogenolysis will not occur, further exacerbating any hypoglycemia!

Results in hepatomegaly and enlarged kidneys secondary to glycogen deposits, and hypoglycemia

↑ G-6-P yields ⊕ Glycogen synthase

Disease	Defect	Effect	S & S, Comments
Type II (Pompe)	lack of α-glucosidase (lysosomal maltase)	reduced access to glucose or glucose-1-PO$_4$ from glycogen, and causes accumulation of glycogen	1. hepatomegaly, cardiomegaly with heart failure, muscle hypotonia, and damage to most other organs 2. death by age 2
Type III (Cori's)	debranching enzyme deficiency	accumulation of all branch points of glycogen	1. hepatomegaly

can utilize all glucose that is not branched

Disease	Defect	Effect	S & S, Comments
Type V (McArdle)	skeletal muscle phosphorylase deficiency	accumulation of glycogen in skeletal muscle	1. McArdle→Muscle 2. when glycogen is needed (exercise), muscle pain and cramps occur with <u>no rise in lactate</u> (a by-product of glycolysis), meaning the muscles are "starved" for glucose for glycolysis 3. progressive muscle weakness, despite muscles having increased glycogen content

glycogen

not enough serum glucose

glucose

glycolysis

pyruvate →LDH→ lactate

Krebs neg feedback

↓O₂

exercise

only step requiring O₂ [e⁻ transport pathway

Section 60.0 — GLYCOSAMINOGLYCANS

GLYCOSAMINOGLYCANS = GAGs = MUCOPOLYSACCHARIDES

- = large complexes of (-) charged heteropolysaccharide chains that can bind large amounts of water to form a gel-like matrix
- comprised of repeating disaccharides, and one of those 2 sugars is always N-acetyl-glucosamine.
- stabilize & support cellular & fibrous components, and maintain water balance of body
- all are "compressible", like a sponge

Types of Glycosaminoglycans

Hyaluronic acid	only GAG that is also in bacteria	Lubricant & shock absorber In synovial fluid, vitreous humor, umbilical cord, & loose CT
Heparin	↑ antithrombin III	Intracellular component of mast cells that line arteries; especially in liver, lung & skin
Keratin SO_4		In cartilage & cornea
Chondroitin SO_4	most abundant GAG	In cartilage, tendons, ligaments, aorta
Dermatan SO_4		In skin, blood vessels, heart Valves
Heparan SO_4	exclusively an extracellular GAG	In bone marrow & is on most cell surfaces as part of the glycocalyx

Section 60.1   MUCOPOLYSACCHARIDOSES

Mucopolysaccharidoses are diseases marked by an inability to metabolize or degrade certain mucopolysaccharides (glycosaminoglycans). The result is the accumulation of excess amounts of certain mucopolysaccharides. They are all due to dysfunction of lysosomes, the cellular component responsible for turn-over and degradation of mucopolysaccharides.

all have accumulation in connective tissue

	defect	result	S&S, comments
Hurler	α-L iduronidase	accumulation of heparan SO_4 & dermatan SO_4	**corneal clouding** **MR/ID** myocardial ischemia (because of deposits in coronary arteries), coarse facial features (gargoyle-like), dwarfing
	different mutations	*different ratios of accumulation*	
Scheie	α-L iduronidase	accumulation of heparan SO_4 & dermatan SO_4	**corneal clouding** **NORMAL intelligence** aortic valve disease stiff joints
		different ratios of accumulation	
Hunter	iduronate sulfatase	accumulation of heparan SO_4 & dermatan SO_4	**NO corneal clouding** **MR/ID** various physical deformities

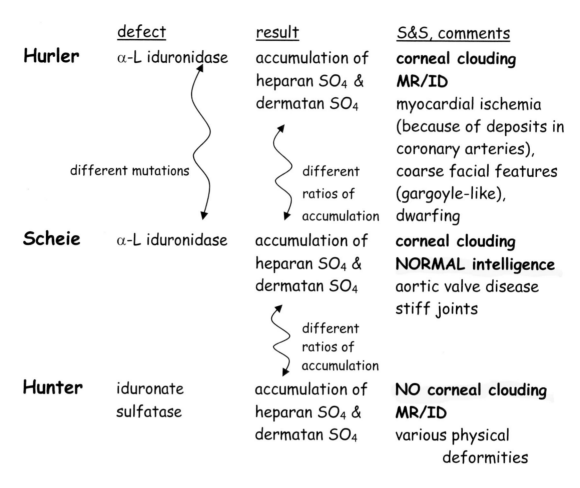

Section 61.0   PROTEOGLYCANS
-lubricants, extra-cellular matrix, molecular sieve

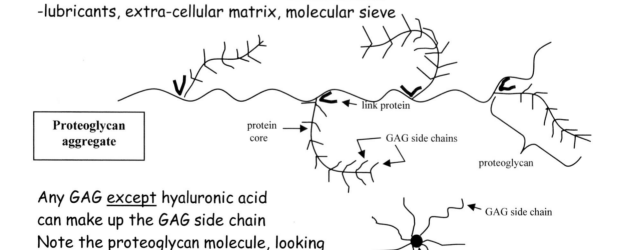

Proteoglycan aggregate

link protein

protein core

GAG side chains

proteoglycan

Any GAG <u>except</u> hyaluronic acid can make up the GAG side chain
Note the proteoglycan molecule, looking at it longitudinally (Bottle Brush model):

GAG side chain

protein core

Proteoglycan: Bottle Brush model

441

Section 62.0   PORPHYRIAS

Porphyrias = defects in heme biosynthesis
- all are AD (except for those that are acquired and
congenital erythropoietic porphyria → AR)

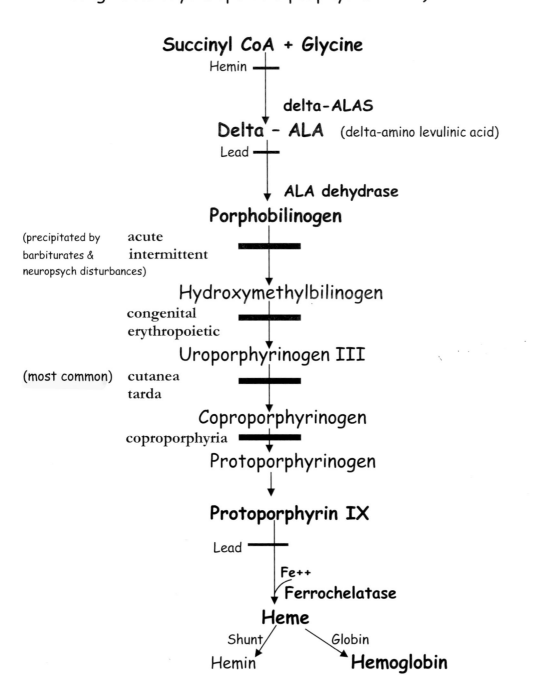

Succinyl CoA + Glycine

Hemin ——|

↓ **delta-ALAS**

Delta – ALA   (delta-amino levulinic acid)

Lead ——|

↓ **ALA dehydrase**

Porphobilinogen

(precipitated by   **acute**
barbiturates &   **intermittent**
neuropsych disturbances)

Hydroxymethylbilinogen

**congenital
erythropoietic**

Uroporphyrinogen III

(most common)   **cutanea
tarda**

Coproporphyrinogen

coproporphyria

Protoporphyrinogen

↓

Protoporphyrin IX

Lead ——|

↓ Fe++
Ferrochelatase

Heme

Shunt ↙   Globin ↘

Hemin   **Hemoglobin**

Porphyrias

1. (+) Photosensitivity if a porphyrinogen accumulates (therefore, acute intermittent doesn't cause photosensitivity since only porphobilinogen, which is NOT a porphyrinogen, accumulates)
2. Microcytic anemia ↓ hemoglobin
3. Abdominal Pain, generalized
4. Oxidative damage to multiple tissues secondary to oxidation of the excess heme precursors; often results in severe cosmetic and functional deformities

Vampires

- sharp teeth
- pale due to anemia
- avoided sunlight
- drank blood to replace heme

Treatment:

1) IV hemin (to slow heme synthesis process, minimizing the likelihood of precursor build-up)
2) avoid sunlight – unless acute intermittent
3) beta-carotene (free radical scavenger that is the best anti-oxidant for hypoxic tissues)

Mechanism of Photosensitivity

Porphyrinogens

Light ∿∿∿→ |

Porphyrins
↓
O_2 ⟶ O_2 radicals → skin damage

Section 63.0 <u>PREFERRED FUELS</u>

<u>Brain</u>

Normally, the brain uses glucose as its sole energy source. However, during the fasting state, it will rely upon both ketone bodies and glucose, with preference for glucose.

<u>Red Blood Cells (Erythrocytes)</u>

RBCs rely on glucose exclusively at any time, whether it is the fed or fasting state.   *RBC only use glucose*

<u>Cardiac Muscle</u>

The heart will use a variety of energy sources, and does so in both the fed and fasting state. In either state, therefore, it will use glucose, lactic acid, ketone bodies, and/or fatty acids. All metabolism in the heart is aerobic, requiring adequate oxygen availability at all times.

<u>Skeletal Muscle</u>

In the fed state, skeletal muscle will rely on different energy sources, depending on whether it is exercising or at rest. At rest, it relies solely on fatty acids. Conversely, while at exercise, it will rely, additionally, on glucose; that glucose is delivered to the muscle by the blood and is also provided via glycogenolysis in the skeletal muscle itself.

Alternatively, skeletal muscle in the fasting state relies on fatty acids, ketone bodies, glucose, and amino acids; among these, the muscle preferentially uses fatty acids.

Skeletal muscle usually functions aerobically, requiring oxygen to carry out metabolism. However, at times of exercise in which inadequate amounts of oxygen are delivered, skeletal muscle has the ability to function anaerobically.

Section 64.0   GLUCOSE & KETONE BODIES: FACTS

Some Facts About Glucose and Ketone Bodies
- During fasting, it is the liver that plays the primary role of maintaining normoglycemia (normal serum glucose levels). It accomplishes this by carrying out glycogenolysis (breakdown of glycogen) and gluconeogenesis (de novo manufacture of glucose).
- Gluconeogenesis, the process of glucose manufacture, requires lactic acid or glycerol or alpha-ketoacids as substrates. The lactic acid is produced by muscle functioning anaerobically (exercising); it is also produced by RBCs continually. Glycerol, on the other hand, is derived from the hydrolysis of triglycerides in adipocytes. Lastly, alpha-ketoacids are derived from the metabolism of glycogenic amino acids (includes all amino acids except tyrosine, phenylalanine, tryptophan, leucine, isoleucine, and lysine).
- Ketone bodies are a metabolite of triglyceride and fatty acid metabolism.

During starvation:
(1) Glycogen stores are exhausted in 10-18 hours (via glycogenolysis).
(2) Gluconeogenesis (creation of glucose from lactic acid, amino acid, fatty acid) begins in 4-6 hours.
(3) After a few days, the rate of fatty acid breakdown exceeds capacity of energy producing processes, yielding increased ketone bodies.

+++

Section 65.0 <u>VITAMINS</u>

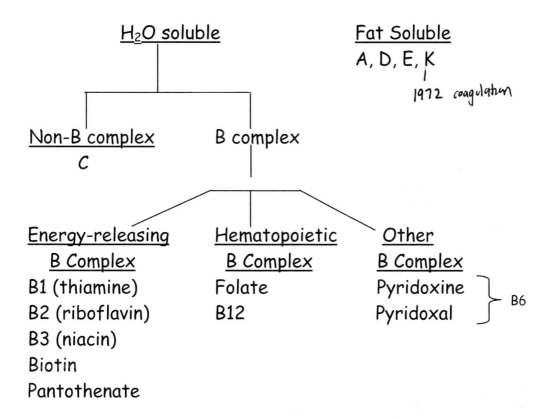

<u>H₂O soluble</u>

<u>Fat Soluble</u>
A, D, E, K
|
1972 *coagulation*

<u>Non-B complex</u>
C

<u>B complex</u>

<u>Energy-releasing B Complex</u>
B1 (thiamine)
B2 (riboflavin)
B3 (niacin)
Biotin
Pantothenate

<u>Hematopoietic B Complex</u>
Folate
B12

<u>Other B Complex</u>
Pyridoxine } B6
Pyridoxal

<u>vitamin</u>	<u>deficiency state</u>	<u>comments</u>
A (retinal) Is part of rhodopsin Needed for normal epithelium Needed for bone growth Needed to maintain fetus	1. Night blindness 2. Skin disorders (acne Tx = retinoic acid) 3. Resorption of fetus 4. Growth retardation 5. Loss of taste	+TOXIC at high doses
C (ascorbic acid) Hydroxylation of proline & lysine for collagen synthesis; antioxidant; cofactor for norepi synthesis	1. Scurvy (sore, spongy gums; loose teeth; fragile blood vessels)	+Prevents CAD +Excellent antioxidant

vitamin	deficiency state	comments
E antioxidant	1. Ataxia 2. Hemolysis in infants	+In vegetable oils +Decreases CAD incidence, decreases LDL, slows Alzheimer's progression
K carboxylation of glutamate → maturation of clotting Factors II, VII, IX, X	1. Bleeding disorder	+Elderly bruise easily partly because of vitamin K deficiency secondary to decreased gut flora +Toxic at high doses→ causes hemolytic anemia +Primarily from bacteria in gut; also in cabbage, cauliflower, broccoli, liver, egg yolk

D
GI tract: Ca absorption
Bone: provision of Ca & P
So, is critical to GI and bone function
	1. Rickets (kids)
	2. Osteomalacia (adults)
	3. Increased risk for:
	    Osteoporosis
	    Colon cancer
	    Pancreatic cancer
	    Breast cancer
	    Type I & Type II DM
	    Higher autism rates
	    MS relapse rates
	    Autoimmune dz
		+TOXIC at high doses (the most toxic of all vitamins) → deposits pathologic levels of Ca^{++} in arteries and kidneys, and VERY high doses increase cancer risk
		+Decreases rate of cellular proliferation
		+Increases rate of apoptosis
		+Decreases renin synthesis, decreasing BP
		+Increases insulin production, aiding glycemic control
		+Acts as a (+) inotrope
		+Found in dairy Products, and formed with exposure to sunshine

447

vitamin	deficiency state	comments

B1
(thiamine)
Decarboxylations
for energy production

1. Beriberi

Wet ———— Dry

Cardiomyopathy

Dry skin;
Disordered thinking:
Irritability

+Found in pork, grains,
legumes

2. Wernicke's encephalopathy
(ataxia, nystagmus, delirium/confusion,
6th cranial nerve palsy)
3. Korsakoff dementia
(severe memory loss, apathy,
impaired thinking)
4. Korsakoff psychosis
(psychosis usually recalcitrant
to anti-psychotics)
5. Infantile deficiency
(convulsions & death of
breast fed infants of
thiamine-deficient moms)

B2
(riboflavin).
FAD, FMN, etc.

1. Glossitis
2. Cheilosis

+found in milk, eggs,
liver, green leafies

B6
(pyridoxine ← plants)
(pyridoxal ← animals)

1. Microcytic anemia

+TOXIC (even though
water-soluble) at high
doses→ neuropathy
+Isoniazid causes B6
depletion
+B6 supplement needed
for high protein diets
+B6 supplementation also
highly recommended for
women on OCPs since they
also mildly deplete B6

vitamin	deficiency state	comments
B12 (cyanocobalamin) Needed for methionine synthesis, DNA synthesis, and odd carbon FA degradation	1. Macrocytic anemia 2. Neuropathy (due to abnormal FA accumulation in neurons)	+ The fish tapeworm *(Diphyllobothrium latum)* consumes B12 in the human gut +Found in eggs, oysters, and liver
B3 (niacin) NADP, NAD	1. Pellagra (dermatitis; diarrhea, dementia → then death)	+ A treatment for hyperlipidemia → increases serum HDL, decreases serum LDL, VLDL, and triglycerides +Inhibits lipolysis
Pantothenate CoA	1. Headache & nausea	+ Found in eggs, liver and yeast
Biotin Carboxylations	1. Nausea and anorexia 2. Seborrheic dermatitis 3. Nervous disorders	+ In almost all food + Avidin (in raw egg white) binds biotin → ingest 20 eggs/day to cause the deficiency
Folic Acid Needed for one carbon metabolism; DNA synthesis	1. Macrocytic anemia 2. Glossitis 3. Colitis 4. Neural tube defects (if mom deficient during 1st few weeks of pregnancy)	+ The most common vitamin deficiency in US → usually seen in alcoholics and pregnant women + ALL sexually active woman of child-bearing age should take 0.4 mg/day of folate!!!

449

Section 66.0   GLYCOLYSIS

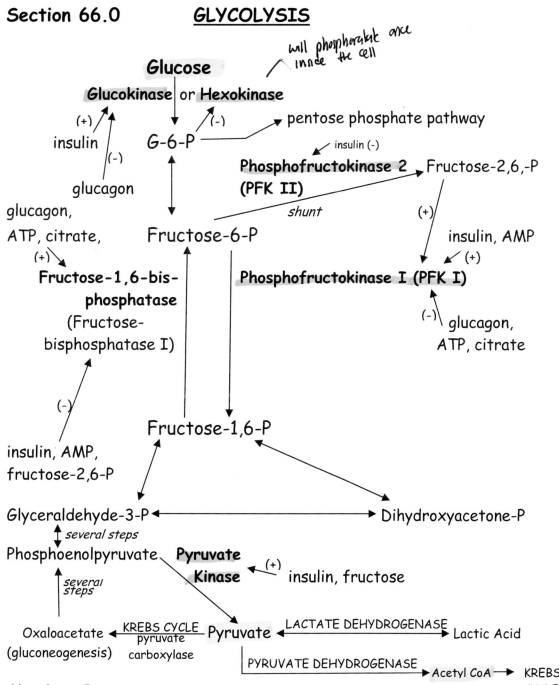

will phosphorylate once inside the cell

Glycolysis Facts:

Glycolysis is the initial metabolic process for glucose to undertake. An excess of fructose-6-P causes activation of PFK II; the product of PFK II (fructose-2,6-P) is a potent activator of PFK I. Another potent activator of PFK I is insulin. When PFK I is activated, more fructose-6-P is metabolized to fructose-1,6-P, thereby causing an increase in glycolytic activity.

Notes:

Section 67.0   GLUCONEOGENESIS

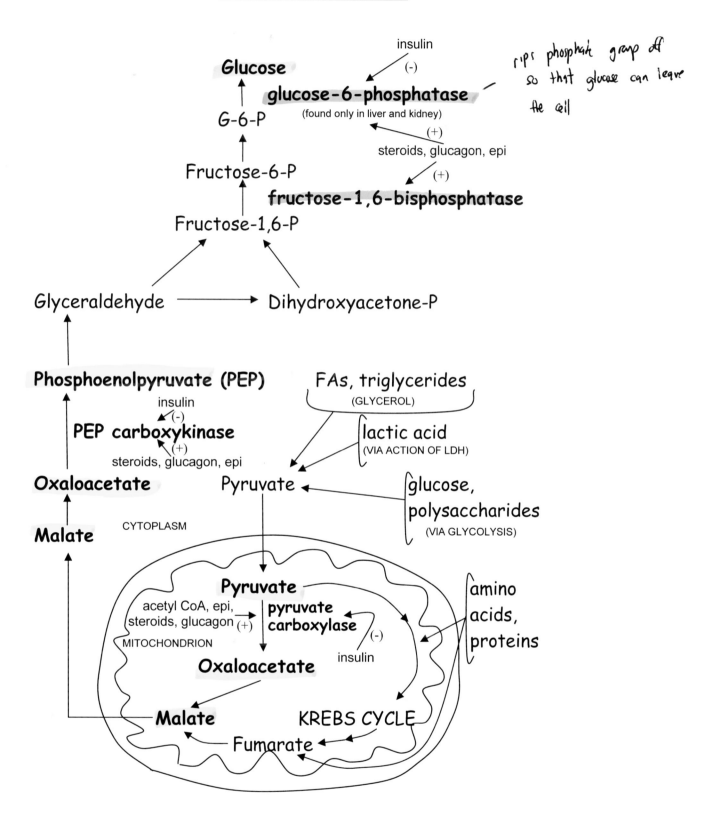

insulin
(-)

Glucose

glucose-6-phosphatase

rips phosphate group off
so that glucose can leave
the cell

G-6-P

(found only in liver and kidney)

(+)
steroids, glucagon, epi

Fructose-6-P

(+)

fructose-1,6-bisphosphatase

Fructose-1,6-P

Glyceraldehyde ⟶ Dihydroxyacetone-P

Phosphoenolpyruvate (PEP)

FAs, triglycerides
(GLYCEROL)

insulin
(-)

PEP carboxykinase

(+)
steroids, glucagon, epi

lactic acid
(VIA ACTION OF LDH)

Oxaloacetate   Pyruvate

glucose,
polysaccharides
(VIA GLYCOLYSIS)

Malate   CYTOPLASM

Pyruvate

acetyl CoA, epi,
steroids, glucagon (+)

**pyruvate
carboxylase**

amino
acids,
proteins

MITOCHONDRION

(-)
insulin

Oxaloacetate

Malate   KREBS CYCLE

Fumarate

GLUCONEOGENESIS FACTS

- Gluconeogenesis is the de novo formation of glucose from alpha-ketoacids derived from glucogenic amino acids (which are, themselves, from free amino acids and proteins), glycerol (from fatty acids, triglycerides), and lactate (from glucose and polysaccharides); other sources include all glycolysis intermediates and all TCA cycle intermediates.

- The glucogenic amino acids include all nonessential amino acids (alanine, arginine, asparagine, aspartate, cysteine, glutamate, glutamine, glycine, proline, serine, and tyrosine) plus all essential amino acids except leucine and lysine (methionine, threonine, valine, isoleucine, phenylalanine, histidine, and tryptophan).

- Gluconeogenesis provides glucose when carbohydrate is not available from the diet; this is especially important since a continuous supply of glucose is necessary for RBCs and the CNS.

- Gluconeogenesis is stimulated by glucagon, steroids (glucocorticoids), and epinephrine, and inhibited by insulin.

- Pharmacologic administration of steroids can cause hyperglycemia because of the activation of gluconeogenic mechanisms.

- The 4 key enzymes for gluconeogenesis are pyruvate carboxylase (which converts pyruvate to oxaloacetate), phosphoenolpyruvate carboxykinase (which converts oxaloacetate to phosphoenolpyruvate (PEP)), fructose-1,6-bisphosphatase (which converts fructose-1,6-bisphosphate to fructose 6-phosphate), and glucose-6-phosphatase (which converts glucose-6-phosphate to glucose which is then free to diffuse out of the cell into the bloodstream).

453

Section 68.0 FATTY ACID SYNTHESIS RATE CONTROL

The rate controlling step of FA synthesis is catalyzed by **acetyl CoA carboxylase.**

Section 69.0 KETONE BODY SYNTHESIS: REVIEW

In **mitochondrion** of liver:

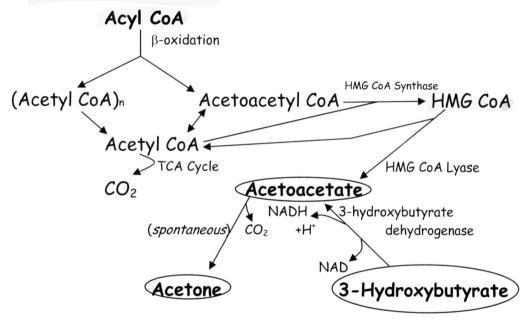

Acyl CoA, derived from fatty acid metabolism, enters the mitochondrion. Upon entry, it is beta-oxidized, a process that removes a two-carbon fragment progressively and repeatedly from the carboxyl end of the acyl CoA. The products yielded from this process are a number of acetyl CoAs (2-carbon molecules), NADH, and $FADH_2$. Under normal circumstances, the acetyl CoA enters the TCA cycle to produce CO_2 and ATP, while NADH and $FADH_2$ enter the electron transport chain to yield ATP. Beta-oxidation unleashes massive quantities of ATP; for instance, palmitoyl CoA (a 16 carbon molecule) generates a total of 131 ATP molecules. If overwhelming amounts of acyl CoA enter the mitochondrion, the TCA cycle is saturated and acetoacetyl CoA, a precursor to ketone bodies, is made.

454

It should be noted that acyl CoA enters the mitochondrion via the assistance of carnitine palmitoyl transferase (also known as carnitine acyltransferase). However, short- and medium-chain fatty acids (e.g., those < 12 carbons long) can enter the mitochondrion without the assistance of carnitine palmitoyl transferase. Because their full metabolism and, ultimately, oxidation is not inhibited by malonyl CoA (malonyl CoA, a product of fatty acid synthesis, inhibits palmitoyl carnitine transferase), short- and medium-chain fatty acids are more readily and more quickly metabolized and less likely to be stored in adipose tissue. Human breast milk and coconut oil are rich in medium-chain fatty acids.

Boards Boot Camp High-Yield Compendium

Section 70.0   PURINE SYNTHESIS

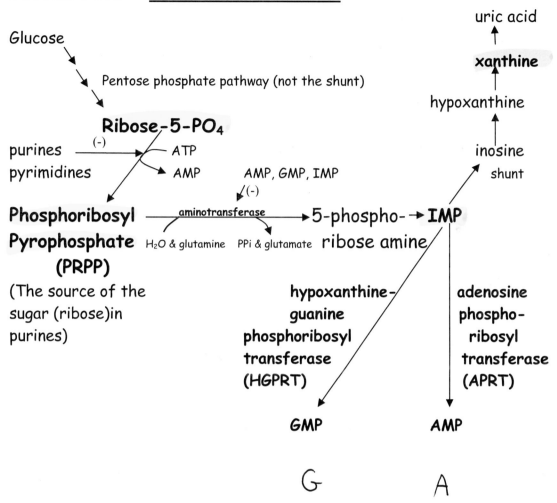

Glucose

Pentose phosphate pathway (not the shunt)

Ribose-5-PO$_4$

purines $\xrightarrow{(-)}$ ATP
pyrimidines   AMP

AMP, GMP, IMP
$\downarrow (-)$

Phosphoribosyl $\xrightarrow{\text{aminotransferase}}$ **5-phospho-** → **IMP**
Pyrophosphate H$_2$O & glutamine   PPi & glutamate **ribose amine**
(PRPP)

(The source of the
sugar (ribose) in
purines)

uric acid
↑
xanthine
↑
hypoxanthine
↑
inosine   shunt

hypoxanthine-   **adenosine**
guanine   **phospho-**
phosphoribosyl   **ribosyl**
transferase   **transferase**
(HGPRT)   **(APRT)**

GMP   AMP

G   A

Section 71.0   PYRIMIDINE SYNTHESIS

Carbamoyl aspartate→orotic acid →OMP→UMP→UDP→UTP→CTP
                                        ↓1-Carbon
                                        ↓Metabolism
                                    dTMP

Section 72.0   CITRIC ACID CYCLE

= KREBS CYCLE = TRICARBOXYLIC ACID CYCLE = TCA CYCLE

Krebs Cycle

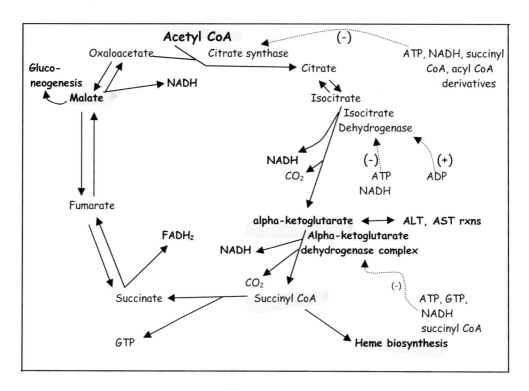

Acetyl CoA is derived from pyruvate; pyruvate dehydrogenase catalyzes this reaction.

Boards Boot Camp High-Yield Compendium

Section 73.0   ATP PRODUCTION: Overview

GLYCOLYSIS → KREBS CYCLE → ELECTRON TRANSPORT CHAIN
(cellular respiration)

Glycolysis Net Products: 2 ATPs (4 are made, but 2 are used)
+ 2 NADHs + 2 Pyruvates
ATP Total = 2 ATPs per glucose

Decarboxylation of Glycolysis End-Product: The glycolysis end-product is pyruvate. It must be decarboxylated to become acetyl CoA, the substrate contributed from glycolysis to the Krebs cycle. Each decarboxylation yields 1 NADH; but, there are 2 pyruvates to be decarboxylated for each glucose that undergoes glycolysis, yielding 2 NADHs total. **ATP Total = 0**

<u>Krebs Cycle (TCA Cycle) Net Products:</u>

Each pyruvate (and 2 are provided from each glycolytic cycle) yields 1 ATP (or GTP) + 1 $FADH_2$ + 3 NADHs
ATP Total = 2 ATPs per glucose

<u>Electron Transport Chain Net Products:</u>

The NADHs and $FADH_2$s that enter from glycolysis, pyruvate decarboxylation, and the TCA cycle yield ATP; each NADH yields about 3 ATPs. Each $FADH_2$ yields 2 ATPs. Thus, for EACH glucose metabolized:

(2 NADH from glycolysis + 2 NADH from pyruvate decarboxylation + 6 NADH from Krebs) + (2 $FADH_2$ from Krebs)
EQUALS
[(2 x 3) + (2 X 3) + (6 x 3) ATPs] + [2 x 2 ATPs]
EQUALS
[6 + 6 + 18 ATPs] + [4 ATPs]

Boards Boot Camp High-Yield Compendium

EQUALS
[30 ATPs] + [4 ATPs]
EQUALS
34 ATPS from electron transport chain from one glucose

ATP Total for Metabolism of 1 Glucose = 34 from electron transport chain + 2 from Krebs + 2 from glycolysis =
38 ATPS (max under optimal conditions)

Section 74.0   Pyruvate Decarboxylation

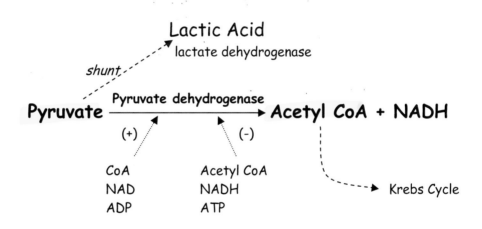

This reaction is necessary to allow the product of glycolysis (pyruvate) to become acetyl CoA so that it can enter the Krebs Cycle.

The NADH that is produced is also used in the electron transport chain to yield about 3 ATPs.

Section 75.0   ENDOCRINE CONTROL OF METABOLISM

Insulin   Secreted by pancreatic β-islet cells
Increased by glucose, amino acids, secretin;
      decreased by epinephrine
Primary role is to make available substrate
      accessible to tissues for metabolism or
      storage

Glucagon   Secreted by pancreatic α cells
Decreased by glucose, insulin; increased by
      hypoglycemia, amino acids, epinephrine
Primary role is to prevent hypoglycemia

Section 76.0   Hormones, Fuels, and Metabolism

MOLECULE	FAT	CARBOs/SUGAR	PROTEIN
INSULIN	ANABOLISM 1. Increases glucose transport into adipocytes 2. Increases lipoprotein lipase activity 3. Inhibits hormone sensitive lipase	ANABOLISM 1. Increases uptake into skeletal muscle & adipose by increasing the number of glucose transporters 2. Increases glycolysis in liver & muscle 3. Increases glycogenesis in liver and muscle	ANABOLISM 1. Increases amino acid uptake
GLUCAGON	CATABOLISM 1. Increases hepatic breakdown of FA 2. Increases ketone body synthesis 3. No effect (or <u>little</u>) on adipose	CATABOLISM & ANABOLISM 1. Increases liver gluconeogenesis 2. Increases liver glycogenolysis 3. No effect on muscle	ANABOLISM 1. Increases amino acid uptake in liver for gluconeogenesis
GROWTH HORMONE	CATABOLISM 1. Increases lipolysis 2. Increases ketogenesis	CATABOLISM & ANABOLISM 1. Increases liver gluconeogenesis 2. Decreases glucose uptake in many tissues	ANABOLISM 1. Increases protein synthesis 2. Increases insulin synthesis (but reduces insulin sensitivity)
CORTISOL	CATABOLISM 1. Increases lipolysis 2. Increases lipogenesis in central body	ANABOLISM 1. Decreases glucose uptake in muscle, adipose 2. Increases liver gluconeogenesis 3. Increases liver glycogenesis	CATABOLISM 1. Increases peripheral protein catabolism 2. Increases hepatic uptake of amino acids

461

Section 76.1   A Note on Epinephrine

Think fight or flight...
Epinephrine causes everything needed metabolically for fight or flight:
Increased lipolysis (for energy)
Increased muscle uptake of glucose (to run or fight)
Increased liver gluconeogenesis (for a ready supply of glucose for energy)
Increased liver & muscle glycogenolysis (for a ready supply of glucose for
energy)

Section 77.0   NUCLEOTIDES

Nucleic acids, namely RNA and DNA, are comprised of nucleotides. Nucleotides
contain nitrogenous bases; there are two types – purines and pyrimidines.

PURINES
Adenine
Guanine

PYRIMIDINES

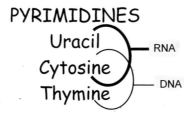

Uracil — RNA
Cytosine
Thymine — DNA

- In **DNA**, Adenine (A) pairs with Thymine (T); Guanine (G) pairs with $A\top$ $C\,G$
  Cytosine (C)
- **RNA** replaces T with Uracil (U) $A\cup$ $c\,G$
- **Codons** are 3 adjacent nucleotides in RNA or DNA
- A DNA codon can contain A, T, G, or C
- An RNA codon can contain A, U, G, or C
- An **anticodon** is 3 adjacent nucleotides in **tRNA** (5'-3') that pair, in the
  opposite direction, with the mRNA codon (3'-5'). So, a tRNA anticodon
  of GAA can pair with an mRNA codon of CUU.
- The **wobble base** is the third codon position in the mRNA. At this
  position, base pairing that is not consistent with Watson-Crick base pair
  rules can occur. At the wobble position, tRNA G can pair with mRNA C
  or U, tRNA U can pair with A or G, and tRNA I (inosine) can pair with
  mRNA A, U, or C. Thus, tRNA of UAC can pair with mRNA GUA or
  GUG.

462

Salvage of Purine Bases

Hypoxanthine $\xrightarrow{\text{HGPRT}}$ **IMP**

Guanine $\xrightarrow{\text{HGPRT}}$ **GMP**

Adenine $\xrightarrow{\text{APRT}}$ **AMP**

Degradation of Purine Bases

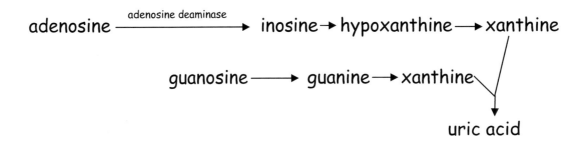

Section 78.0   <u>SOME BASICS: Transcription & Translation</u>

DNA = deoxyribonucleic acid; it is present in the nucleus and in mitochondria

RNA = ribonucleic acid; there are several types:

mRNA =	messenger RNA; it is the product of transcription (copying) of a DNA strand. mRNA is what determines the amino acid sequence of proteins to be produced.
tRNA =	transfer RNA; it is the molecule that transports certain amino acids to the ribosome for use in protein manufacture (translation).
rRNA =	ribosomal RNA; it is intimately involved with the structure of the ribosome
Transcription =	the process of "reading" a DNA strand to produce an RNA strand (mRNA)

Translation =	the process of "reading" mRNA to determine the amino acid sequence of a growing polypeptide (protein); occurs at the ribosome

Section 78.1   <u>TRANSCRIPTION</u>

DNA → RNA
Catalyzed by RNA polymerase

<u>Bacteria (Prokaryotes)</u>
Holoenzyme = core enzyme + σ factor
Holoenzyme means Whole Enzyme, and acts as the RNA polymerase used in bacteria

("whole enzyme")	core enzyme → it is responsible for 5'-3' RNA polymerase activity; it is non-specific and cannot recognize promoter region of DNA
	σ factor →does recognize the promoter region; binds to core enzyme, allowing RNA polymerase recognition of promoters
Cistron	region of DNA that encodes a single protein

*Prokaryotic mRNA is polycistronic (encodes multiple proteins) as opposed to human (or any eukaryotic) mRNA which only codes for one protein.

Notes:

Boards Boot Camp High-Yield Compendium

Human (Eukaryotic)

HUMAN (Eukaryote) Promoter

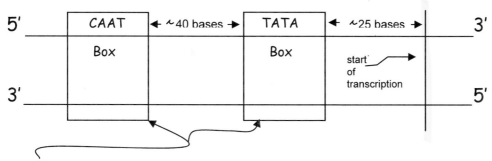

Sequences recognized by **RNA Polymerase II** in the eukaryotic promoter region

Enhancers are regulatory DNA Sequences. They bind with enhancer binding proteins that interact with transcription factors bound to a promoter. **Transcription factors** bind to the **TATA box**, and are necessary for **RNA polymerase** recognition of the promoter region.

There are 3 types of RNA polymerases:

Polymerase I   makes rRNA (more specifically,
                                     precursors of large rRNA → 28s,
                                     18s, 5.8s in nucleolus)

Polymerase II   makes mRNA, which is later transcribed
                                     into protein
                              inhibited by alpha-amanitin (remember,
                                     a potent toxin from poison
                                     mushrooms and toadstools)

Polymerase III   makes tRNA (and 5s rRNA)

RNA PROCESSING

Eukaryotic mRNA is heavily processed in the nucleus <u>after</u> its formation but BEFORE it leaves the nucleus:

1. **5'-cap** (methylated GTP) is added; 7-methyl-guanosine is attached backwards to the 5' terminal end of mRNA.

   5'-cap **facilitates initiation of translation and helps to stabilize mRNA.**

2. **Poly-A tail** is added to the 3' end. Poly-A tail is not transcribed from DNA, but added via a nuclear enzyme known as Poly-A polymerase. The tail **helps mRNA exit from nucleus and helps stabilize mRNA.** (mRNA does not exit until all processing is completed).

3. **Introns** are removed and **exons** (remaining mRNA material) are **spliced** together.

   snRNA (small nuclear RNAs (produced primarily by polymerase II)) and proteins join to from **snRNPs** (small ribonucleoprotein particles). snRNPs bind to the ends of introns, bringing together neighboring exons into correct alignment for splicing. This results in excision of introns.

Section 78.2   <u>DNA REPLICATION</u>

Eukaryotes

DNA polymerases cannot initiate synthesis of a new DNA strand but require an RNA primer (short oligonucleotide sequence composed of RNA, made by RNA primase). The primer is later replaced by DNA.

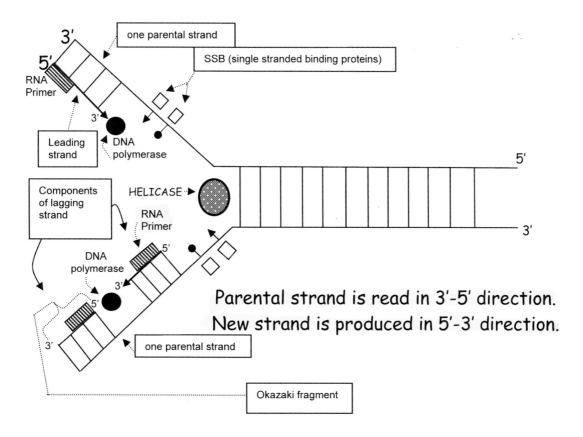

Parental strand is read in 3'-5' direction.
New strand is produced in 5'-3' direction.

<u>Dna A Protein</u> = binds to specific nucleotide sequences at AT rich sites, causing strands to melt apart leaving 2 strands

<u>SSB</u> = single stranded binding proteins; bind to ssDNA after helicase acts. These serve to prevent re-annealing.

<u>Helicase</u> = binds to single strands, and separates parental dsDNA.

<u>Primase</u> = an RNA polymerase that copies parental strand and makes RNA primer → makes short RNA that remains bound to ssDNA that was its template; a DNA polymerase recognizes this configuration and takes over where primase leaves off.

<u>Ligase</u> = joins Okazaki fragments to form lagging strand

EUKARYOTIC DNA POLYMERASES

Pol α   is the RNA primase

Pol β   performs DNA repair via base excision and filling of gaps in the strand

Pol γ   replicates and repairs the DNA; has 3'-5' exonuclease proofreading ability

Pol ε   proofreads via 3'-'5' exonuclease activity, and is thought to continue the primer elongation on the leading strand

Pol δ   proofreads via 3'-5' exonuclease activity, and is thought to continue the primer elongation on the lagging strand

No human DNA polymerases remove the primer; that is performed by non-polymerase enzymes

BACTERIAL (PROKARYOTIC) DNA POLYMERASES

Polymerase I   <u>unlike</u> polymerase II & III; it can remove nucleotides that are correctly base-paired but represent the primer. So, polymerase I removes nucleotides from the primer in a 5' to 3' direction (acting as a "5' exonuclease", and, operating in a direction opposite to all other polymerases!) & replaces those ribonucleotides with deoxyribonucleotides. Hence, RNA primer is replaced with DNA.

Polymerase II   DNA repair enzyme because it has 3' exonuclease activity

Polymerase III   THE major DNA polymerase
copies both parental strands, and only reads & copies parental strands in 3' to 5' direction
has proofreading ability & 3' exonuclease activity to remove wrong nucleotides

----

Humans vs. Bacteria:

1) Replication in human cells is much slower than that in bacteria:
   In Eukaryotes → 100 nucleotides/sec
   In Prokaryotes → 1000 nucleotides/sec

2) Replication occurs at MANY origins of replication in human cells, whereas replication occurs in only one origin of replication in each bacterium.

PHYSIOLOGY

Section 79.0   Intracellular vs. Extracellular Components

- Extracellular fluid has a high sodium concentration, high calcium concentration, and a low potassium concentration; the opposite is true of the intracellular environment.

- Phosphates and proteins are present in higher concentrations within the cell than they are in the extracellular environment.

- The intracellular region is separated from the extracellular environment by the **cell membrane**. Cell membranes are comprised of a bilayer (double layer) of phospholipids. Attached to or buried within this **phospholipid bilayer** are proteins. **Integral proteins** are buried within the membrane, and extend the entire thickness of the membrane. **Peripheral proteins** are on the surface of the membrane, either the internal or the external surface. These two types of membrane proteins play important roles:

Roles of Membrane Proteins

Type of Membrane Protein	Role(s)
INTEGRAL PROTEINS	**Ion channels/pores** (for diffusion) **Carrier proteins** (for facilitated transport or for active transport) **Enzymes**
PERIPHERAL PROTEINS	**Hormone receptors**

- The entire outside surface of most cells is also coated in a carbohydrate mesh known as the glycocalyx

Major Roles of Glycocalyx
1) Aids in cell-to-cell attachment
2) Acts as "receptor substances" (facilitating the attraction of some hormones, such as insulin, to the cell surface to ensure higher likelihood of hormone binding to its actual receptor on the cell surface)
3) Aids with nutrient attachment and eventual absorption via villi of bowel

- Many organelles ("organs of the cell," such as endoplasmic reticulum, nucleus, etc.) are also bounded by a plasma membrane comprised of a phospholipid bilayer.

Section 80.0   Transport through the Cell Membrane

Transport through the cell membrane occurs by way of:
DIFFUSION or ACTIVE TRANSPORT

- Some transport can occur directly through the phospholipid bilayer of the cell membrane. Other transport requires a carrier protein or an ion channel.

- Most carrier proteins are free-floating integral proteins of the cell, and so allow for the passage of substances from the intracellular to extracellular environment, or vice versa. Occasionally, however, they can be part of intercellular connections, whereby they allow for passage of substances from the intracellular environment of one cell to the intracellular environment of another.

There are 2 types of intercellular connections:
1) Tight junctions (zonula occludens)
2) Gap junctions

Tight junctions are attachments that exist between some cells. They sometimes may act as a pathway for certain solutes of a particular size, charge, or shape to pass directly from one cell to another.

Gap junctions are attachments between cells that always allow passage of current and/or ions from one cell to another.

471

Section 80.1   <u>DIFFUSION</u>

- Diffusion occurs either directly through the phospholipid bilayer (for hydrophobic substances and water) or through ion channels or pores (for hydrophilic substances).

<u>There are 2 types of diffusion</u>: **simple diffusion and facilitated transport**

There are 2 types of **simple diffusion**:

1) diffusion down a concentration gradient (e.g., from an area of high concentration to an area of low concentration) directly through the cell membrane
Example: water (osmosis) and small lipid-soluble molecules

   Note: Osmosis = flow of water down *its* concentration gradient, moving from an area of low solute particle number (therefore, "high" water concentration) to an area of high solute particle number.

2) diffusion down a concentration gradient directly through a channel in the membrane
Examples: <u>voltage gated channels</u> (e.g. sodium channels that open to allow passage of sodium; they open when the inside of the cell membrane loses its negative charge (a voltage change), thereby allowing an influx of sodium into the cell when the channel opens) AND <u>chemical gated channels</u> (also known as ligand gated; the channels open when a molecule not intended for cell entry binds to the channel, allowing the passage of a different type of molecule or ion; for example, acetylcholine binds to channels, allowing for sodium entry)

Facilitated transport requires a carrier protein that will bind to the substance to be transported; this channel allows for shuttling or movement of this molecule across the membrane without the use of energy.

- is also known as carrier mediated diffusion

- involves 2 steps:
1) the molecule to be transported enters into a dead-end channel in the carrier molecule, and binds to that carrier molecule
2) the binding allows for a conformational change of the carrier molecule (channel) such that the channel no longer is dead-ended and actually allows for movement of the formerly bound molecule to the other side of the membrane

- glucose and amino acids can cross cell membranes via this mode in some cell types, e.g., simple glucose carriers (such as on the basolateral membrane of gut cells)

Boards Boot Camp High-Yield Compendium

Section 80.2   ACTIVE TRANSPORT

* moves substance against an electrochemical gradient, using energy in the process
* is executed via carrier proteins
* there are 2 types of active transport:

1)   **primary active transport** - the energy is derived from ATP or similar phosphorylated molecules

   Examples of primary active transport:

   Na-K pump *(transports 3 sodium ions out of cell for every 2 potassium ions pumped in, regardless of intra- and extra-cellular concentrations)*

   H/K ATPase *(the "proton pump") - found in gastric parietal cells and in the collecting duct of the kidney; works to pump hydrogen ions into the stomach or into the renal tubule, and, for each hydrogen ion (proton) pumped, a potassium ion is pumped in the opposite direction.*

   Ca-ATPase *(the "calcium pump") - found on the sarcoplasmic reticulum and works to pump calcium back into the sarcoplasmic reticulum from the cytoplasm*

2)   **secondary active transport** - the energy is obtained from energy stored in the form of concentration differences of ions across a cell membrane; that original ion gradient was established by primary active transport. Thus, the transport of the second ion is "coupled" to the transport of the original (different) ion, making this "coupled transport."

There are 2 types of secondary active transport: **Cotransport and Countertransport**

CO-TRANSPORT, e.g. the Na-K pump establishes a significant Na ion gradient, with one side of the cell membrane having a significantly higher Na concentration than the other. Then, a carrier protein that is not related to the Na-K pump allows Na free passage, allowing it to move from an area of high concentration to an area of low concentration (remember, the initial concentration gradient was established by, indeed, the Na-K pump). The diffusion energy stored and created as the Na ions rush through that second carrier protein can facilitate the movement of other molecules with the Na but against their own gradients.

For example, glucose and amino acids can enter certain cells by way of co-transport:

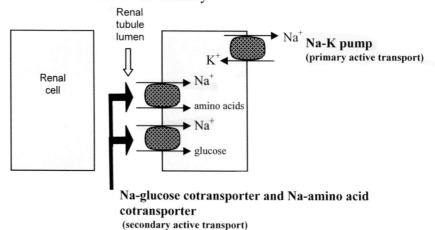

Proximal Convoluted Tubule of the Kidney

Secondary active transport

The diagram above depicts how a primary active transport (Na-K pump in this case) causes a gradient (lowered intracellular Na concentration in this case), that allows for the movement of an ion (Na in this case) down its concentration gradient (with respect to the Na cotransporters in this case) and, via the concentration gradient and the energy from that, the movement of other molecules against their concentration gradient (glucose and amino acids in this case). This is cotransport because the Na is moving in the same direction as the glucose and amino acids via the cotransporter.

475

COUNTER-TRANSPORT, e.g. the Na-K pump establishes a significant Na ion gradient, with one side of the cell membrane having a significantly higher Na concentration than the other. A specially configured carrier protein, different than the Na-K pump, allows Na free passage, allowing it to move from an area of high concentration to an area of low concentration. The diffusion energy stored and created as the Na ions rush in is translated by this carrier protein to allow for passage of a different ion or molecule in the opposite direction of the Na movement.

For example, calcium is transported out of the cell via a sodium counter-transport mechanism; many cell membranes undertake this process (using the "Na-Ca counter-transporter"). Also, hydrogen ions (protons) are transported into the lumen of the proximal convoluted tubule of the kidney via this counter-transport mechanism, whereby Na enters the PCT cells.

Section 81.0   ION CHANNELS

- are integral proteins
- are selective, allowing only certain ions to pass across the membrane
- responsible for the action potential
- they may be open or closed; if open, the ions for which they are selective will pass freely down their concentration gradient

- ➢ the more the ion channel is open, the more ions can permeate the cell membrane. Hence, "permeability" is determined by the probability of the ion channel being open.
- ➢ **Permeability** is also known as **conductance**

- whether an ion channel is open or closed is determined by gates. There are 2 types of ion channels based on the type of gates they have:

  1) **voltage-gated channels** (changes in membrane potential across the cell membrane)

  - ➢ membrane potential (in mV) of any ion is calculated via the Nernst equation:
    $$E = +/- 60mV \log_{10} ([I]/[E])$$
    where I equals intracellular concentration of a particular ion and E equals the extracellular concentration at 37 degrees Celsius (this is not a COMLEX required equation)*
  - ➢ membrane potential is the voltage difference between the outside of the cell and the inside of the cell

- ➢ voltage is created by the separation of electrical charges, via the charges on ions, across a resistive barrier, the cell membrane being the barrier in this case
- ➢ so voltage is created by differences in ion concentration and total charge differences between the inside of the cell and the outside of the cell
- ➢ when the concentration of ions and the total charge of the inside or outside of the cell changes, that changes the voltage. That changes the membrane potential, and that either opens or closes certain ion channels.
- ➢ an example includes the Na channel that allows for the action potential

2) **ligand-gated channels** (binding of neurotransmitters, hormones, or second messengers to the ion channel causes it to open or close)

➢ binding of a neurotransmitter, hormone, or second messenger to the channel causes it to undergo a conformational change that allows the ion for which it is selective to free flow down its concentration gradient across the cell membrane

Boards Boot Camp High-Yield Compendium

❖ The Nernst equation calculates the potential inside the membrane, and provides an arbitrary value for what the potential of that particular ion would be to enter the cell. At rest, a (+) potential is assigned to a negative ion, and a (-) potential is assigned to a positive ion. The larger the value of the potential, the greater the likelihood for that ion to enter the cell, and the greater the difference in concentration of that ion between the inside and outside of the cell at rest.

> ➤ an example includes the acetylcholine receptor; when acetylcholine binds to it, it allows for Na entry into the cell. The acetylcholine receptor is actually a ligand-gated ion channel.

The Action Potential

1) The membrane is at its resting membrane potential (approximately – 70mV in most cells, approximately – 90mV in neurons)

Inside cell:
lots of K^+

2) A negative value for membrane potential implies that the inside of the cell is more negative than the outside of the cell

3) Small inward currents, such as influx of small amounts of sodium ions (such as what occurs through the ACh receptor), cause a change in the membrane potential (remember, membrane potential = the difference in electrolyte concentrations and in charges between the intracellular and extracellular environment; accordingly, any inward entry of sodium ions will cause a change in membrane potential).

Boards Boot Camp High-Yield Compendium

4) As small amounts of Na⁺ enter the cell, the resting membrane potential becomes less negative (remember, the larger the value of the resting membrane potential, the greater the difference in concentration of that ion between the inside and the outside of the cell. During rest, the sodium concentration is much greater extracellularly than intracellularly. As more sodium enters, that "difference" between the two sides of the cell membrane decreases; thus, the membrane potential decreases in VALUE. So, the membrane potential will move from, for nerves, -90 mV to, let's say, -80 mV. The value of the potential decreases (e.g., the difference decreases).

5) Eventually, as more and more Na⁺ enters, the membrane potential becomes depolarized; literally, <u>depolarization</u> means to remove (de-) any differences (polarize). So, by reducing the difference in Na concentration between the inside and the outside of the cell, the cell has been depolarized.

6) Eventually, the cell, if it is a neuron, reaches – 70 mV to – 50 mV. At this voltage, the neuron has reached its "threshold to activation" and the cell can now propagate an action potential.

7) Depolarization to the threshold causes a rapid conformational change in the Na channels (ion channels specific to sodium ions).

8) As a result to the conformational change, there is rapid opening of the activation gates of the **Na** channels

9)   This causes rapid, overwhelming increased **Na** influx

10)   Depolarization also closes the inactivation gates of the **Na** channels (but more slowly than it opens the activation gates)

11)   Depolarization also slowly opens **K** channels, increasing **K** conductance (K movement across the cell membrane)

12)   This increased potassium ion conductance results in significantly increased **K** efflux (greater than that at rest)

13)   The Na^+ conductance, with sodium ions entering, remains higher than the K^+ conductance, with potassium ions leaving.

14)   So much Na^+ quickly enters that the sodium equilibrium potential becomes $+65$ mV, meaning that a point is reached in which there is no longer any potential for the sodium to enter and that the inside of the cell has become positive.

15)   The process of changing the potential not only goes from negative to 0, but then progresses to a high positive value; that means that overshoot has occurred.

16)   The inactivation gates of the Na channels eventually close, blocking any further sodium movement through those channels.

17) The conductance of **K** remains high much longer after the closure of the **Na** channels, driving the membrane potential towards the **K** equilibrium potential

18) So, now that all Na channels are closed, the now-open K channels take the lead in the process; the rapid exit of potassium ions (which are positively charged) causes the inside of the cell to lose positive charge, bringing it closer to a negative value.

19) As the membrane potential becomes more negative, it starts to re-establish its resting membrane potential; this process is known as repolarization.

20) However, since the potassium ions stay open so long while the Na channels are still immobilized, potassium leaks out of the cell to the point of establishing almost its own membrane potential.

21) The K^+ equilibrium potential (the potential it naturally assumes by itself with a cell) is much more negative than the resting membrane potential.

22) Thus, the membrane potential assumes a potential much more negative than usual; this is known as undershoot, or positive afterpotential (although it is negative), or hyperpolarization

23) Eventually, the K^+ channels become less conductive

24) The cell regains its resting membrane potential

Boards Boot Camp High-Yield Compendium

The Action Potential

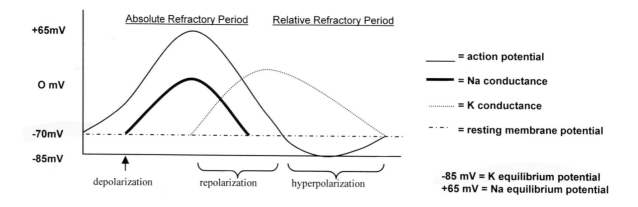

Absolute refractory period – due to closure of **Na** inactivation gates; once they close, they will not reopen until the resting membrane potential or greater polarization than that is attained. Until then, it is impossible to have any Na entry. Thus, it represents a period of time in which another action potential cannot be generated.

Relative refractory period – occurs during hyperpolarization. To generate an action potential during this period, a stronger than usual stimulus is needed to counter the higher **K** efflux (the hyperpolarization)

483

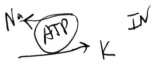

out ... Na ← ATP → K ... IN

K channels - maintains resting membrane potential because **K** has a very high permeability (conductance). That is why the resting membrane potential is so close to the **K** equilibrium potential.

Na channels - at rest, these are closed.
- repolarization is due to closure of inactivation gates of **Na** channels.

Ca channels   EXCITATION CONTRACTION COUPLING: excited muscle releases **Ca** from **SR** (sarcoplasmic reticulum). **Ca** attaches to troponin C which pulls tropomyosin off the myosin binding site, therefore triggering contraction.

Cl Channels   CNS: INHIBITORY POSTSYNAPTIC POTENTIALS   Inhibitory synapses open Cl instead of Na channels on post-synaptic neuron, allowing for chloride ion entry. Also, pre-synaptically, GABA is released by inhibitory neurons onto presynaptic bulb, increasing Cl influx into the presynaptic bulb; the result is hyperpolarization and a state of relative refraction to any action potential.

Na/K Pump - maintain ion gradient (3 Na out of every 2 K in); therefore, creates a net negative charge on the inside of the cell. However, has only a small contribution to overall resting membrane potential – remember, most of that potential is contributed by potassium's equilibrium potential.

Section 81.1 Neurophysiology

❖ **Action potentials** that travel from the periphery to the CNS represent **afferent** impulses; those that travel from the CNS to the periphery represent **efferent** impulses.

❖ There are several different nerve fiber types:

Fiber Type	Example	Size	Conduction velocity
A-alpha	α-motoneuron	largest	fastest
A-beta	touch afferents	medium	medium
A-delta	pain afferents	small	medium
A-gamma	γ-motoneuron to muscle spindles	medium	medium
B	pre-ganglionic fibers of the autonomic nervous system (ANS)	small	medium
C	post-ganglionic fibers of the ANS	smallest	slowest

❖ Neuronal impulses are transmitted in the following manner:

1. As the **action potential** reaches the end of the presynaptic neuron (the neuron before the synapse), it causes calcium ions to enter the terminal bulb (the end) through Ca^+ channels

2. **Calcium entry** into the presynaptic terminal bulb causes the bulb to release, through exocytosis, a neurotransmitter into the synapse (synaptic cleft; the space between the end of the presynaptic neuron and the beginning of the postsynaptic neuron).

3. The **neurotransmitter** diffuses across the synapse to the surface of the post-synaptic neuron where it binds to receptors.

4. Inhibitory neurotransmitters hyperpolarize the post-synaptic membrane while excitatory neurotransmitters depolarize the post-synaptic membrane.

5. The post-synaptic cell integrates all inhibitory and excitatory input.

❖ **Excitatory neurotransmitters** cause depolarization (via Na^+ and K^+ channels) and, therefore, bring the post-synaptic cell closer to an action potential. Examples of neurotransmitters that can be excitatory include:

Acetylcholine
Epinephrine
Norepinephrine
Glutamate
Serotonin
Dopamine

❖ **Inhibitory neurotransmitters** hyperpolarize the cell (via chloride channels) and, therefore, bring the cell further away from an action potential. Inhibitory neurotransmitters include:

GABA (gamma-aminobutyric acid)
Glycine

❖ Each neurotransmitter binds to its own receptor on the post-synaptic cell membrane:

Neurotransmitter	Receptor
Acetylcholine	Cholinergic – allows Na entry
Norepinephrine	Adrenergic receptor effect varies by specific type of adrenergic receptor
Epinephrine	Same as for norepinephrine
Dopamine	Dopamine receptors (D1 receptors activate adenylate cyclase and D2 receptors inhibit adenylate cyclase; adenylate cyclase inhibition causes decreased Ca entry while adenylate cyclase activation increases Ca entry in the terminal bulb of the presynaptic neuron)
Serotonin	5-HT receptors (different types have different effects)
Histamine	Histamine receptors (e.g., H1, H2)

487

Glutamate	Kainate receptor – acts a Na^+ and K^+ ion channel
Glycine	Glycine receptor (that increases Cl^- conduction)
GABA	GABA receptors ($GABA_A$ increases Cl^- conduction and is the site of action of barbiturates and benzodiazepines; $GABA_B$ increases potassium permeability); both are highly inhibitory

❖ Neurotransmitters in the synapse are eventually removed from the synapse
  ➢ The catecholamines (epinephrine, norepinephrine, and dopamine) are metabolized by monoamine oxidase (MAO) and catechol-O-methyltransferase (COMT)

Locations of Neurotransmitters

NEUROTRANSMITTER	PRIMARY LOCATION
Acetylcholine	many areas of brain, but primarily is secreted by large pyramidal cells of the motor cortex, different neurons of the basal ganglia, motor neurons of the peripheral nervous system, post-ganglionic nerve fibers of the parasympathetic nervous system, all preganglionic nerve fibers of the autonomic nervous system, and post-ganglionic sympathetic nerve fibers to the sweat glands and piloerector muscles. In the CNS, it is an excitatory neurotransmitter, but in some peripheral locations, it acts as an inhibitory neurotransmitter.
Norepinephrine	secreted by many neurons that originate in the hypothalamus and brainstem, especially the norepinephrine-secreting neurons of the locus ceruleus in the pons (these neurons have long axons that reach large expanses of brain and that, through norepinephrine, serve to aid in control of activity levels and states of wakefulness).
Epinephrine	secreted only by the adrenal gland, but is released to the bloodstream to have systemic effects; it works as an excitatory neurotransmitter

Boards Boot Camp High-Yield Compendium

Dopamine	secreted by neurons that originate in the substantia nigra and that innervate the striatal region of the basal ganglia; it usually works as an inhibitory neurotransmitter there
Serotonin	secreted by neurons that originate in the median raphe of the brain stem and that innervate many areas of the brain and spinal cord, most especially the hypothalamus and the dorsal horns of the spinal cord. It works to inhibit pain pathways in the spinal cord, and to help to control mood. It acts as either an excitatory or inhibitory neurotransmitter, depending on the 5-HT receptor involved.
Glutamate	secreted by extensive areas of the cerebral cortex, and is also secreted by many neurons in the sensory pathways
Glycine	secreted throughout the spinal cord and acts as an inhibitory neurotransmitter
GABA	secreted throughout the cerebral cortex, the spinal cord, the cerebellum, and the basal ganglia; acts as an inhibitory neurotransmitter

---

Boards Boot Camp High-Yield Compendium

Section 82.0   <u>AUTONOMIC NERVOUS SYSTEM</u>

= sympathetic nervous system (SNS) + parasympathetic nervous system (PNS)

Sympathetic preganglionic nerve fibers leave the spinal cord via all of the thoracic nerves and the first two lumbar nerves (L1 and L2). (Remember, there is no sympathetic nervous contribution that emanates out of any area below L2). They then synapse with **sympathetic post-ganglionic neurons (ganglia)** in the **sympathetic chain**. The neuronal processes of the sympathetic post-ganglionic neurons then extend all the way to the tissues to receive sympathetic stimulation.

Parasympathetic preganglionic nerve fibers include those fibers that are carried by **cranial nerves III, VII, IX, and X, as well as via sacral nerve roots S2, 3, and 4** that combine to form the pelvic splanchnic nerves. These preganglionic nerve fibers extend all the way to the tissue to be parasympathetically innervated, and then synapse with a **post-ganglionic neuron**. It is the fibers that extend from that post-ganglionic neuron that then directly innervate the tissue.

The neurotransmitter released by all (SNS and PNS) preganglionic nerve fibers to stimulate the post-ganglion nerve is **<u>ACETYLCHOLINE</u>**.

The neurotransmitter released by all PNS postganglionic nerve fibers to innervate the tissues is **<u>ACETYLCHOLINE</u>**.

The neurotransmitter released by most SNS post-ganglionic nerve fibers is **NOREPINEPHRINE**. There are 2 exceptions:

1) Sweat glands and piloerector muscles are innervated by the sympathetic nervous system; however, the neurotransmitter released by these SNS post-ganglionic nerve fibers is **ACETYLCHOLINE**. These are considered "cholinergic sympathetic fibers."

2) Adrenal medulla is essentially a tangle of post-ganglionic neurons. When it is stimulated by preganglionic sympathetic nerve fibers, it in turn releases **NOREPINEPHRINE and EPINEPHRINE**.

ACETYLCHOLINE is also used in one other peripheral nervous system location other than those situations involving the autonomic nervous system:

The **NEUROMUSCULAR JUNCTION**

Presynaptic motor neurons, after calcium entry into their terminal bulbs, release acetylcholine into the neuromuscular junction which, in turn, stimulates skeletal muscle.

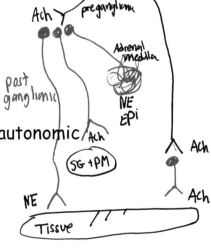

Section 82.1
NEUROTRANSMITTERS and THEIR RECEPTORS

There are 2 types of receptors associated with the autonomic nervous system:
1)   cholinergic receptors
2)   adrenergic receptors

Cholinergic Receptors – bind acetylcholine

They are found on skeletal muscle, on all post-ganglion neurons (both SNS and PNS), and on all parasympathetically innervated tissues

ACh

There are 2 categories of cholinergic receptors:

1) **Muscarinic Receptors** — the type on all parasympathetically innervated tissues

2) **Nicotinic Receptors** — there are two types:

Type I nicotinic receptors – found on all post-ganglionic neurons (both SNS and PNS)

Type II nicotinic receptors – the type of receptor on all skeletal muscle

Adrenergic Receptors – bind norepinephrine and epinephrine

There are 4 types of adrenergic receptors:

1) **Beta Receptors** – there are two types:

493

Beta One Receptors - bind norepinephrine and epinephrine with equal efficacy
- found on cardiac muscle tissue, juxtaglomerular — ↑renin cells, beta islet cells, and adipocytes

Beta Two Receptors - bind epinephrine much more strongly than norepinephrine
- found on coronary arteries, hepatocytes, gallbladder and bile ducts, bronchi, uterus, and blood vessels within skeletal muscle

2) **Alpha Receptors** – there are two types:

Alpha One Receptors - bind epinephrine slightly better than norepinephrine
- found on dozens of different tissues throughout the body

Alpha Two Receptors - found on beta islet cells, platelets, presynaptic nerve bulbs of SNS and CNS

494

Section 82.1.1 <u>MUSCARINIC RECEPTORS</u>

These are postsynaptic PNS receptors; ACh (acetylcholine) binds them.

These are a type of cholinergic receptor.

The other type of cholinergic receptor is the nicotinic cholinergic receptor. Nicotinic cholinergic receptors are ligand gated channels that, when bound by their ligand (ACh), allow Na to flow into the cell; they are the receptors of ALL autonomic ganglia, the adrenal medulla, and the neuromuscular junction.

Muscarinic Receptors:

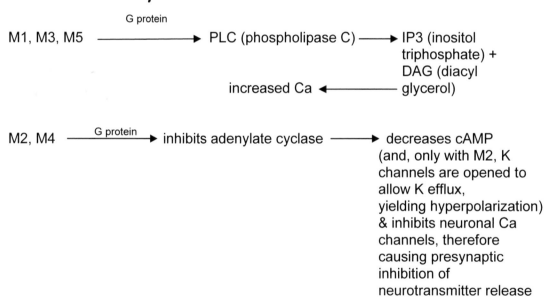

<u>The types of G proteins</u>:
   Gq   activates PLC (phospholipase C)
   Gi   inhibits adenylate cyclase
   Gs   stimulates adenylate cyclase
   Go   inhibits neuronal Ca channels

Boards Boot Camp High-Yield Compendium

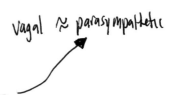
vagal ≈ parasympathetic

Muscarinic Receptors

	G protein	Receptor	Target Organ
stimulatory muscle	Gq	**M1**	**gastric parietal**, vascular smooth (very limited), ANS ganglia, brain
inhibitory	Go & Gi	**M2**	**heart**
stimulatory	Gq	**M3**	**exocrine glands, ALL smooth muscle except vascular (bronchial, GI/GU), vasculature** (which is stimulated to produce NO (nitric oxide) yielding vasodilatation), **many organs**
inhibitory	Go	**M4**	CNS
stimulatory	Gq	**M5**	CNS

M3 is the MAJOR receptor in terms of numbers. It has effects in many areas:

eye...miosis, ciliary muscle contraction
lung...bronchoconstriction, increased secretions
GI/GU...increased motility, increased secretions, bladder/detrusor contraction, sphincter relaxation *"M3 makes you PEE"*

Section 82.1.2 ADRENERGIC RECEPTORS *Sympathetic*

Post-ganglionic sympathetic nerve fibers are all adrenergic, EXCEPT those to sweat glands (as well as piloerector muscles and a few blood vessels). In all cases that are exceptions, these areas are innervated by neurons that emanate from the SNS but that release ACh instead of NE.

Adrenergic Receptors

Receptor	G Protein	Target Organ EFFECTS
alpha 1	Gq	*via post-synaptic SNS:* mydriasis, trigone & sphincter contraction, decreased salivary secretion, decreased nasal secretion, **GI inhibition, vasoconstriction** *via adrenal medullary epinephrine release:* increased sweat gland secretion (mostly on palms and soles) plus piloerection (sweat glands and piloerectors are physically innervated by cholinergic sympathetics and so normally are stimulated by acetylcholine via cholinergic receptors, unless under extreme stress wherein epinephrine from the adrenal medulla adds stimulation via alpha 1 receptors)
alpha 2	Gi	*via presynaptic SNS & CNS:* ?venodilation, GI relaxation, **decreased insulin release, increased coagulation** (alpha 2 is on platelets → decreased cAMP → Na-H exchange → Ca influx → arachidonic acid pathway → thromboxane produced → platelet aggregation)
beta 1	Gs	*via post-synaptic SNS:* **heart, kidney** (via juxtaglomerular cells, causing renin release), adipocytes (generating lipolysis)
beta 2	Gs	*via post-synaptic SNS:* **vasodilatation of blood vessels in skeletal and cardiac muscle, bronchodilatation**

THE SNS (sympathetic nervous system) neurotransmitter = NE!!! (except for the adrenal medulla…from which NE &, especially, **Epi** are released to the blood stream for <u>RAPID, SYSTEMIC, BODY-WIDE</u> effects)

NT	ALPHA-1	BETA-1	BETA-2	
NE	++++	++	++	primary effect is vasoconstriction….therefore, increased DBP (diastolic blood pressure) (Beta 1 effect yields moderate SBP (systolic blood pressure) increase)
Epi	+++++	++	++++	primary effect is vasodilatation in skeletal muscle….therefore, decreased DBP (Beta 1 effect yields moderate SBP increase)
Isoproterenol	+	++++	++++	primary effect is extreme skeletal muscle vasodilatation with extreme heart stimulation…therefore, increased SBP with very decreased DBP

NT = neurotransmitter
NE = norepinephrine
Epi = epinephrine

497

Section 82.2 AUTONOMIC NERVOUS SYSTEM EFFECTS
= PNS & SNS effects

Most tissues are dominantly controlled by either the PNS or SNS.

Response is determined by which receptors are present in highest numbers.

Site	Sympathetic	Parasympathetic
Coronary arteries	dilated (β2) constricted (better shunting)(alpha 1)	dilated (M3)
Apocrine glands	thick, odiferous secretion (alpha 1)	none
Lung blood vessels	mildly constricted (alpha1)	?dilated (M3)
Liver	glucose release (β2)	slight glycogen synthesis (M3)
Gallbladder & Bile Duct	relaxed (β2)	contracted (M3)
Heart	increased rate (β1) increased conductance (β1) increased force of contraction (β1)	decreased rate (M2) decreased force of contraction (especially of atria) (M2)
Bronchi	dilated (β2)	constricted (M3)
GI Tract	decreased motility (alpha 1)	increased motility (M3)
GI Tract Sphincters	constricted (alpha 1)	relaxed (M3)
Rectum	allow filling (alpha 1)	empties (M3) relaxes internal sphincter concomitantly

Site	Sympathetic	Parasympathetic
Bladder	detrusor relaxed (alpha 1) trigone contracted (alpha 1)	detrusor contracted (M3) trigone relaxed (M3)
Erection	none	maintains erection (M3)
Ejaculation	triggers ejaculation (alpha 1)	none
Pupils	mydriasis via contraction of meridonal fibers of iris (alpha 1) re: dilator pupillae	miosis via contraction of circular m. of iris (M3) re: constrictor pupillae
Sweat Glands	cholinergic	none
Salivary glands	vasoconstriction...thick secretion (alpha 1)	vasodilation...copious secretion (M3)
All Glands not already noted (nasal, lacrimal, parotid, sublingual, submandibular, gastric), parietal cells	vasoconstriction & slight thickened secretion (alpha 1)	copious secretion (M3)

The glands of the small and large intestines are controlled primarily by local factors on the intestinal tract itself and by the intestinal enteric nervous system (i.e. innervation by intramural plexus = intestinal enteric nervous system), and much less by the ANS.

Arterioles
1) abdominal viscera constricted (alpha 1)		none
2) muscle	constricted (alpha 1) **dilated** (beta 2)	dilated (very slight) (M3)
3) skin	constricted (alpha 1)	none

Blood
coagulation	increased (alpha 2)	none
glucose & lipids (serum levels)	increased (alpha 2)	none

499

Site	Sympathetic	Parasympathetic
Mental activity	increased (alpha 2)	none
Piloerector mm	cholinergic-contracted	none
Fat cells	lipolysis (β1)	none
Uterus	relaxation (β2)	contracted (M3)

Section 83.0 SIGNAL TRANSDUCTION

Signal transduction refers to how a cell translates ligand binding to that cell into an action undertaken by that cell. Signal transduction, therefore, is initiated by the binding of a ligand, such as a hormone or neurotransmitter, to that cell. The ligand binds to a specific receptor on the cell. Once the ligand is bound to the receptor, it sets a series of reactions into motion within the cell. These reactions are carried out by second messengers. Eventually, the second messengers mediate some action on behalf of the cell. The entire process of ligand binding, second messenger activation, and, ultimately, cellular response is signal transduction.

The 5 Major Second Messenger Systems
1. IP3 mechanism
2. Cyclase mechanism
3. Calcium-calmodulin mechanism
4. Steroid hormone mechanism
5. Tyrosine kinase mechanism

G proteins are used in all second messenger systems except for the steroid hormone mechanism and tyrosine kinase activation. They couple ligand receptors to biochemical responses. They can be either inhibitory or stimulatory. All have three subunits: alpha, beta, and gamma. It is the alpha subunit that determines their inhibitory or stimulatory role.

Notes:

Boards Boot Camp High-Yield Compendium

1. IP3 Mechanism

IP3 = inositol triphosphate
DAG = diacyl glycerol

IP3, DAG – neurotransmitters/hormones bind to a receptor in the cell membrane and, via G protein, activate phospholipase C which liberates DAG & IP3 from membrane lipids. IP3 mobilizes calcium (Ca) from ER (endoplasmic reticulum). Ca and DAG activate protein kinase C (PKC) which phosphorylates proteins, causing specific physiologic reactions.

ligands: *ACh on M1, M3, M5 receptors; NE or Epi on alpha one receptors; histamine on H1 receptor; and TRH, ADH, Oxytocin, GnRH, and GHRH on their respective receptors*

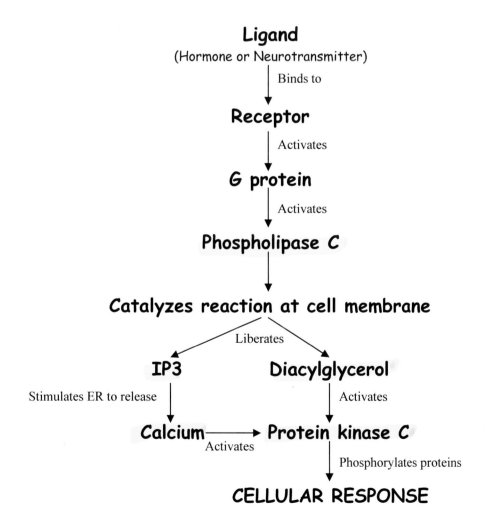

Ligand
(Hormone or Neurotransmitter)

Binds to

Receptor

Activates

G protein

Activates

Phospholipase C

Catalyzes reaction at cell membrane

Liberates

IP3   **Diacylglycerol**

Stimulates ER to release   Activates

Calcium ⟶ **Protein kinase C**

Activates

Phosphorylates proteins

CELLULAR RESPONSE

2. Cyclase mechanism

In this mechanism, a hormone or neurotransmitter binds to its respective receptor on the cell, and that receptor binding triggers the G protein to release a GDP and replace the GDP with a GTP. This now-activated G protein (e.g., loaded with a GTP) either inhibits or activates a cyclase enzyme (adenylate cyclase or guanylate cyclase). The result is either an increase or decrease in cAMP or cGMP levels. Both cAMP and cGMP are able to inhibit or activate very specific metabolic processes.

G Protein Action on Adenylate Cyclase

cAMP - levels determined by adenylate cyclase (& phosphodiesterase). Gi or Gs inhibit or stimulate adenylate cyclase, respectively. Activated adenylate cyclase results in cAMP production which, itself, increases activity of protein kinase A. PKA then phosphorylates key proteins and enzymes to bring about the cellular changes. Inhibited adenylate cyclase has, of course, the opposite effect.

cAMP = cyclic AMP

> NE or Epi on beta 1 receptor....Gs....increased cAMP → increased heart rate and force of contraction
>
> NE or Epi on beta 2 receptor....Gs....increased cAMP → vasodilation in skeletal muscle vasculature and bronchodilation in lungs
>
> histamine on H2 receptor....Gs.....increased cAMP → gastric parietal cells stimulated to increase HCl acid secretion
>
> ACh on M2 or M4 receptor....Gi...decreased cAMP → decreased heart rate and decreased CNS activity
>
> NE or Epi on alpha 2 receptor....Gi....decreased cAMP → decreased sympathetic nervous system activity

Other hormones that bind to a receptor to activate G protein that then mediates control over adenylate cyclase include ACTH, TSH, LH, FSH, PTH, calcitonin, ADH, and glucagon.

Boards Boot Camp High-Yield Compendium

G Protein Action on Guanylate Cyclase

cGMP – levels determined by guanylate cyclase.

cGMP = cyclic GMP

G protein can cause the production of cGMP via activation of guanylate cyclase. In addition, membrane-bound guanylate cyclase can be directly stimulated by ANP. Soluble guanylate cyclase can be directly stimulated by nitric oxide.

EDRF (endothelial derived relaxing factor) – contains the active component, NITRIC OXIDE (NO). EDRF is released by endothelial cells (the cells that comprise the inner lining of blood vessels) when those cells are placed under shear stress. Basal levels are present in healthy people to keep GFR (glomerular filtration rate) and Na excretion high to prevent hypertension (therefore, people without it get HTN). GFR is increased by NO (nitric oxide) because of decreased renal vascular resistance. It is the NO (EDRF) that stimulates guanylate cyclase; the guanylate cyclase then manufactures cGMP which, itself, leads to less cytoplasmic Ca in smooth muscle cells. The decreased cytoplasmic calcium levels occur because cGMP stimulates increased Ca pumping into SR (sarcoplasmic reticulum) and increased pumping of Ca out of cells. The decreased cytoplasmic Ca concentrations result in vascular smooth muscle relaxation, thereby causing vasodilation.

ALSO, NO acts as a neurotransmitter in the brain that is released by pre-synaptic neurons. It does NOT depolarize post-synaptic neurons, but causes internal changes that last minutes, hours, or longer and play a role in memory.

ANP (atrial natriuretic peptide) - from atrial heart muscle, and produced when atria are over-stretched; increases GFR and Na secretion, decreases blood volume, and inhibits renin. These effects occur because ANP causes the stimulation of guanylate cyclase and the resulting production of cGMP.

Phosphodiesterase-5 inhibitors (e.g., sildenafil) – these have no effect on guanylate cyclase, but do inhibit the very enzyme responsible for cGMP degradation. The result is an accumulation of cGMP. The increased cGMP causes vasodilation (due to its effects on cytoplasmic calcium in vascular smooth muscle) of the penile artery with concomitantly improved vascular filling of the penis. This results in erection.

3. Calcium-Calmodulin Mechanism

A ligand (hormone) binds to its respective receptor on a cell and, consequently, activates a G protein. As a result, calcium is mobilized from intracellular stores and calcium is also allowed to enter the cell via opening of calcium channels in the cell membrane. The increased cytoplasmic calcium concentrations increase the likelihood for calcium to bind with calmodulin. Once 3 to 4 of the calcium-binding sites are bound up with calcium, the calmodulin undergoes a conformation change; this conformational change serves to activate a wide variety of enzymes known as calcium/calmodulin-dependent kinases (CaM kinases). One of the most specific roles of calmodulin is to activate myosin light chain kinase, a type of CaM kinase, which then acts on smooth muscle myosin to bring about smooth muscle contraction.

Ligands for this mechanism include those substances that stimulate endothelin receptors and M1 receptors, specifically endothelin and acetylcholine, respectively. Endothelin is released by damaged or traumatized endothelial cells (inner lining of blood vessels), and causes profound local vasoconstriction when bound to endothelin receptors. Acetylcholine binding to M1 receptors causes hydrochloric acid and intrinsic factor release in the stomach to facilitate digestive processes.

4. Steroid Hormone Mechanism

Steroids diffuse through the cell membrane and bind to a receptor in the cytosol (type I nuclear receptor; type I NR) or in the nucleus (type II nuclear receptor; type II NR). Type I NR-steroid complexes enter the nucleus as dimers (couplets). The latter, acting as transcription factors, bind to the steroid-responsive elements (SREs; hormone response elements; HREs) on DNA. The type II NRs exist perpetually in the nucleus, heterodimerized to RXR (retinoid X receptor) on the DNA. When hormone enters the nucleus, it displaces a corepressor on the type II NR, forming an NR-steroid complex that binds to

505

HRE on the DNA and acts as a transcription factor. Regardless of the receptor type, in both cases, DNA transcription is stimulated, causing mRNA to be made and, eventually, protein synthesis to be initiated. These proteins have specific physiologic functions, allowing the cell to transduce the "message" of the steroid into a physiologic action by the cell.

The steroids that function through the steroid hormone mechanism include hormones that bind to Type I NRs (aldosterone, glucocorticoids, testosterone, estrogen, and progesterone) and the hormones that bind to Type II NRs (thyroid hormones and vitamin D).

Note: Recent research has shown some estrogen receptors also reside in the nucleus, too!

5. Tyrosine Kinase Mechanism
When insulin binds to alpha subunits of the insulin receptors, beta subunits are autophosphorylated by tyrosine kinase. The phosphorylated receptor enters the cells and phosphorylates enzymes, bringing about a cellular response to the insulin. Insulin-like growth factor-1 (IGF-1; also known as somatomedin C) has similar effects on this mechanism.

Section 84.0   NYSTAGMUS
Hall Pike Bithermal Caloric Test – performed to assess health of labyrinth:
1.   Patient is supine 30 degrees (to position that places horizontal   semicircular canals in the vertical plane) and eyes straight ahead
2.   Irrigate ear with cold water (86 degrees F)
              - nystagmus should be to opposite irrigated ear
3.   Irrigate ear with warm water
              - nystagmus should be to same ear side

Think COWS --- Cold Opposite, Warm Same (side) --- if this doesn't happen, then there is a dead labyrinth.

Nystagmus direction is determined by to what side the fast movement of the eyes point; so, if the eyes move quickly, repeatedly to the right but slowly back to the left, then that is a right nystagmus.

Boards Boot Camp High-Yield Compendium

2 Classifications of Nystagmus:

1. Pendular
    - Eyes appear to swing back and forth, doing so at equal speed to either side – like a pendulum
    - Due to ocular disorders (e.g., blindness) or pathology at the optic chiasm
2. Jerk
    - Represents the most common type of nystagmus
    - Eyes jerk rapidly and involuntarily
    - There are 2 major movement types:

    (A) VERTICAL

    (B) HORIZONTAL

Vertical Nystagmus
- o The eyes vibrate or move vertically
- o Always represents CNS pathology
- o There are two major vertical nystagmus categories:
    1. Downbeat – the fast phase of movement goes downward in a vertical path; due to typically cervicomedullary lesions. *herniated / cerebellum* Examples of causes include Arnold-Chiari syndrome, as well as CVA or MS of the lower brainstem (medulla)
    2. Upbeat – the fast phase of movement goes upward in a vertical path; due to brainstem and vermis lesions. Causes can include CVA, MS, and tumors.

Horizontal Nystagmus
- o The eyes vibrate or move horizontally
- o Can represent pathology of the CNS or pathology of peripheral structures

o There are 3 major horizontal nystagmus categories:

1. <u>Periodic alternating</u> – the fast phase goes repeatedly to one side horizontally, and then switches after a certain period of time so that the fast phase then goes to the other side horizontally; therefore, this "alternates" sides periodically; it is due to vestibulocerebellar disease (such as CVA, MS, tumors of that region) or due to bilateral visual loss

2. <u>Gaze-evoked</u> – only occurs or is exacerbated when one looks to a particular side; it can be caused by EtOH intoxication or intoxication with other depressants, by cerebellar disease, and by brainstem lesions

3. <u>Vestibular</u> – the fast phase is always to one particular side on a horizontal plane; this can be due to disease of the inner ear, cranial nerve VIII, or the central nuclear complex. It is often accompanied by vertigo, tinnitus, +/- deafness. However, if it is caused by central nuclear complex pathology, the nystagmus may also have a vertical or rotatory component and the vertigo, tinnitus, and/or deafness tend to be milder. Examples of potential causes of vestibular nystagmus are labyrinthitis, Meniere's disease, or ischemia or trauma to the aforementioned regions.

Section 85.0   <u>COCHLEA</u>

Cochlear base: has narrow stiff hairs, making it sensitive to high frequency
                         sound
Cochlear helicotrema: has wide compliant hairs, making it sensitive to low
                             frequency sound

1.   Sound is transmitted through the oval window
2.   The sound waves then move the basilar membrane
3.   Movement of the basilar membrane causes movement of the hair cells
       located on top of the basilar membrane
4.   The movement of the hair cells causes bending of the cilia of the hair
       cells
5.   This all occurs in an oscillating fashion – and ciliary bending one way
       causes increased K conductance while opposite bending causes
       decreased K conductance – hyper- and hypopolarization, causing
       oscillating cochlear microphonic potentials

Section 85.1   **HEARING APPARATUS**
Human Speech = 300-3000 Hz
Tuning Fork to be used: 512 or 1024 Hz

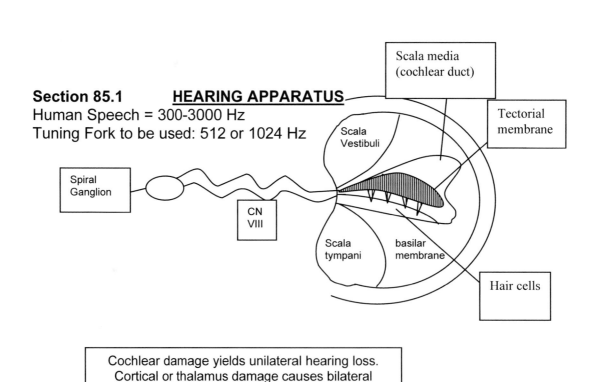

Cochlear damage yields unilateral hearing loss.
Cortical or thalamus damage causes bilateral
hearing loss.

Section 85.2   **TUNING FORK TESTS**

Weber
to determine lateralization

Rinne
to determine air and bone conduction

First, place base of vibrating fork on mastoid process until tone disappears (=bone conduction): place level with canal

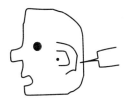

place base of vibrating fork on top of skull or on mid-forehead

Then, quickly hold next to ear (= air conduction); place the U facing anteriorly

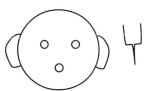

Conductive
ear w/ conductive loss will hear better
- no other externally can distract from tuning fork

Sensineuronal
ear w/ conductive loss will hear less
- not functioning as well

⊖ normal ear can continue to hear thru air after bone
⊕ conductive hearing loss will ↓ sensineuronal hearing
⊕ can continue hearing through air
- works better than conduction even though it has lower function

Hearing Loss: Conductive vs. Sensineuronal

How they compare:

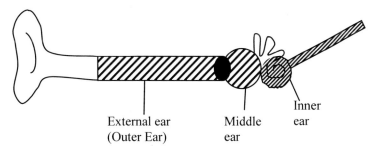

/// = locale of conduction deafness

▨ = nerve (sensineuronal) – cochlear n.

	Conductive	**Sensineuronal**
Causes	OM, eardrum perf, cerumen, obstruction of ear canal	nerve damage (i.e. from sustained exposure to loud noise, drugs, inner ear infections, *aminoglycosides* congenital and hereditary disorders, aging (presbycusis))
Distortion of Sound	minor	distorted with upper tones of words (which are even often LOST)
Noisy environment	hearing improves	hearing worsens
Patient's voice	normal (because still conducted thru bone)	loud (because can't hear self)
Age of Onset	Up to 40, esp. childhood	middle to late years
Weber	lateralized (X) to bad ear b/c not distracted by other sounds	lateralizes (X) to good ear

(handwritten note: otitis media)

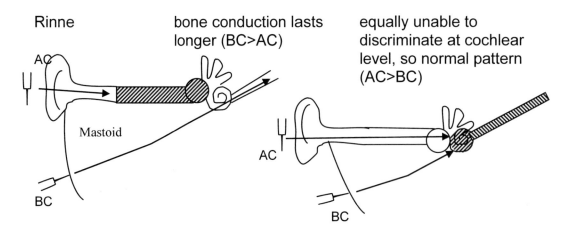

Lateralization means to hear the vibration sound better on one side than the other; when it lateralizes to one side, that means it is heard better on that side as opposed to the other side

	Conductive	**Sensineuronal**
Rinne	bone conduction lasts longer (BC>AC)	equally unable to discriminate at cochlear level, so normal pattern (AC>BC)

AC

Mastoid

BC

AC

BC

Section 86.0   **CONTROL OF MUSCLE TONE**

MUSCLE SPINDLE

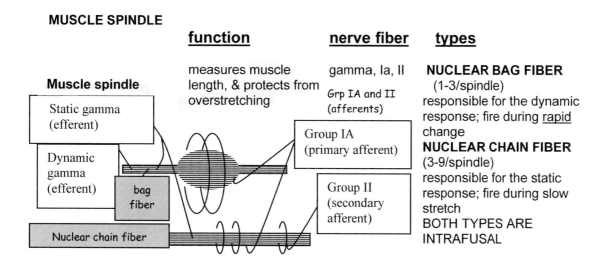

	function	**nerve fiber**	**types**
Muscle spindle	measures muscle length, & protects from overstretching	gamma, Ia, II Grp IA and II (afferents)	**NUCLEAR BAG FIBER** (1-3/spindle) responsible for the dynamic response; fire during <u>rapid</u> change
Static gamma (efferent)		Group IA (primary afferent)	
Dynamic gamma (efferent)		Group II (secondary afferent)	**NUCLEAR CHAIN FIBER** (3-9/spindle) responsible for the static response; fire during slow stretch BOTH TYPES ARE INTRAFUSAL

When skeletal muscles (extrafusals) are overstretched, muscle spindles are stretched. Then, group IA +/- Group II afferents send afferent impulses to the spinal cord; there, they stimulate alpha-motoneurons, causing contraction of that original skeletal muscle (the extrafusal muscle). Muscle spindle fibers are intrafusal muscle fibers. Muscle spindle fibers prevent overstretching of skeletal muscle (and are also responsible for mediating the afferent part of the deep tendon reflex).

GOLGI TENDON ORGAN

	function	**nerve fiber**	**types**
Golgi tendon organ	measures muscle <u>tension</u>, preventing TENDON overstretch. When stimulated, they inhibit A-alpha motoneurons	1B afferents no efferents (because they need not be innervated to "do" something)	all are the same

inhibitory reflex
inhibits agonist and cause an antagonist contraction

Note: The muscle spindle fibers are responsible for all stretch reflexes (deep tendon reflexes; DTRs)

512

Section 87.0   SKELETAL MUSCLE ACTIVATION

Skeletal muscle is innervated by **large, myelinated nerve fibers** that arise from the **motorneurons** in the spinal cord. Each nerve fiber typically stimulates anywhere between **three and several hundred skeletal muscle fibers**; the fewer muscle fibers it innervates, the finer the motor skill imposed. The junction created between the nerve fiber and skeletal muscle is called a **neuromuscular junction.** The nerve fiber contains vesicles containing **acetylcholine**. The acetylcholine in the vesicle is manufactured via enzymatic action of **choline acetyl transferase** on acetyl coenzyme A (CoA) and choline. When an action potential spreads over the cell membrane of the nerve fiber, **calcium channels** open, allowing calcium to diffuse into the nerve fiber terminal. The calcium mobilizes the acetylcholine-filled vesicles to move toward the cell membrane in order to open and release their contents. Therefore, the **acetylcholine is released** via exocytosis from these vesicles, permitting acetylcholine to enter the neuromuscular junction.

Acetylcholine binds to **nicotinic Type II receptors** on skeletal muscle. These receptors are **acetylcholine-gated (chemical gated) ion channels** which, when bound with 2 molecules of acetylcholine, allow for the **diffusion of large numbers of sodium ions** to enter the skeletal muscle cell. The entry of such large numbers of Na ions also imposes the entry of a large number of positive charges into the cell; this causes a potential charge at the muscle fiber membrane at that site. With enough entry, an **action potential** can be created.

Acetylcholine in the neuromuscular junction is eventually destroyed by **acetylcholinesterase.**

There are three types of muscle in the body: smooth, cardiac, and skeletal. There are two types of skeletal: red skeletal and white skeletal.

Type I / Red Skeletal Muscle   *Type II* / White Skeletal Muscle

1 slow red ox

Red Skeletal Muscle	White Skeletal Muscle
slow fibers	fast fibers
posture, marathons, endurance	rapid, powerful…sprints
small muscle	large muscles
low strength	very high strength
low glycolytic ability	high glycolytic ability
high oxidative ability (therefore, rely a lot on electron transport pathway; therefore need high O_2. They have a high # of mitochondria and a hi # of capillaries)	low oxidative ability
low # of glycolytic enzymes	hi # of glycolytic enzymes
high blood supply	low blood supply
high # of mitochondria	low # of mitochondria
low SR (sarcoplasmic reticulum)	very high SR network
primary type of metabolism: oxidative	primary type of metabolism: glycolytic
(+) myoglobin (stores O_2 and imparts red color)	NO myoglobin

All skeletal muscle operates via motor units. One motor unit is the total of ALL muscle fibers (muscle cells) that are innervated by a single alpha-motoneuron. This is different than that of cardiac and smooth muscles, wherein they operate as a syncytium (e.g., due to structures that allow for communication of ions and charge directly between them, stimulation of one cell in the syncytium results in stimulation of all cells of that tissue).

Skeletal muscle contraction is mediated by calcium binding to troponin. The same mechanism occurs in cardiac muscle. However, in smooth muscle, calcium binds calmodulin to bring about MLC phosphorylation.

The calcium that is used by skeletal muscle is derived from calcium released into the cytoplasm from sarcoplasmic reticulum. In cardiac muscle, it is an influx of calcium from outside the cell that is required for contraction to occur. Smooth muscle uses both influx and release methods.

514

Section 87.2   SKELETAL MUSCLE CONTRACTION

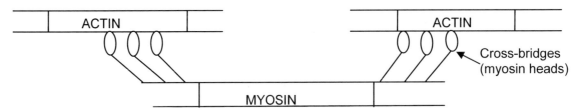

1. Myosin heads bind with ATP
2. The head's intrinsic ATPase activity cleaves ATP...ADP + Pi (both still bound to head)
3. Step 2 forces the head to sit perpendicular toward the actin, but NOT yet attached to the actin:

   > (or it unattaches from actin at this point, if it was attached from the last contraction)

4. Troponin C binds with Ca.
5. Troponin then tugs on tropomyosin, moving away from the actin active sites, exposing the latter.

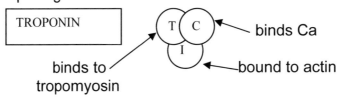

6. Myosin heads bind to actin active sites.

7. Then, the myosin head tilts toward the arm of the crossbridge:

   This is the POWER STROKE (the energy is provided by steps 1 and 2)

8. While the head is still tilted, ADP and Pi are released

9.   A new ATP molecule binds (and the cycle begins again – see #1 and onward)

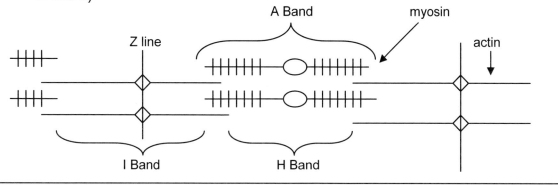

Section 88.0   Pulmonary Physiology

Air is delivered to the lung through the trachea (**first generation respiratory passageway**), then the right and left bronchi (**second generation respiratory passageways**), and then subsequent divisions (that each amount to another generation). There are a total of about 20-25 generations before the air reaches the alveoli. The rate at which new air reaches the alveoli is known as alveolar ventilation. Some of the air that is inspired never reaches the gas exchange areas; this includes air that never goes beyond the nose, or pharynx, etc. This is **dead space air** and the areas they occupy are collectively known as **dead space**.

At the alveolus, carbon dioxide is received from the pulmonary capillaries and exhaled out; concomitantly, oxygen diffuses from the alveolus to the capillary, providing oxygenation of the blood.

Section 88.0.0   Airflow and Airway Resistance

Surfactant decreases alveolar surface tension by decreasing the attraction of water molecules to one another; without surfactant, water molecules on the inner lining of the alveolus are attracted to one another, forcing the alveolar walls to collapse.

Type II pneumocytes produce surfactant.

NOTES:

Surfactant = **lecithin** (primarily) = dipalmitoylphosphatidylcholine = a phospholipid. Fetuses initially produce sphingomyelin that is then replaced gradually by surfactant (lecithin). Generally, any infant at or less than 34 weeks of gestation is at risk of having insufficient lecithin and, therefore, an increased risk for neonatal respiratory distress syndrome; such an infant is said to be premature. Thus, when mothers go into labor at or before the 34th week of gestation, the sphingomyelin and lecithin levels are measured in the amniotic fluid. There should be more than twice as much lecithin as sphingomyelin (e.g., a ratio of > 2:1) for there to be adequate surfactant to maintain open airways.

Smaller **alveoli** have a greater tendency to collapse.

With respect to alveoli, $P = 2t/r$, where P equals pressure (inward, that encourages alveolar collapse), t = surface tension (which is reduced with surfactant), and r equals radius. Thus, the larger the radius or size of the alveolus, the less the tendency to collapse. Likewise, the less surfactant there is, the more surface tension there is, and the more tendency there is for the alveolus to collapse.

Collapse of many alveoli results in **atelectasis**.

The walls of both the bronchi and bronchioles are lined by smooth muscle that is under PNS and SNS control. Sympathetic activation causes bronchial smooth muscle relaxation and, thus, bronchodilation. This is why beta-2 agonists, agents that stimulate a sympathetic response, and anticholinergic agents (such as ipratropium), agents that inhibit the bronchoconstrictive effects of the parasympathetic nervous system, are used with disorders that benefit from decreased airway resistance, such as asthma, COPD, and pneumonia.

Airway resistance can be described by Poiseuille's law, which is expressed as follows:

$R = \eta L8/\pi r^4$
where R = resistance, η = inspired gas viscosity, L = length of airway, and r = radius of airway.

As we can see, airway resistance and resistance to "breathing" increase with increasing length of the airway. However, the effect of that is miniscule compared to the role that the airway radius plays. In fact, the single most important determinant in airway resistance is the diameter of the airway. That means that bronchodilators work to increase "r" (radius) which, in turn, <u>reduces</u> airway resistance to the fourth-power for each increment increase in radius. For instance, if the radius increases by a factor of 5, the resistance will <u>decrease</u> by a factor of 5^4, or 625.

It should also be noted that increased viscosity of the inspired gas also increases airway resistance, making respiration more difficult. Thus, air replete with pollution, airborne particles, or even humidity increases the airway resistance.

Thus, **airflow** is inversely proportional to airway resistance. Airflow can be represented by the following equation:

Q = ΔP/R, where Q = airflow, ΔP = difference in (gradient) of pressure between mouth and alveoli, and R = airway resistance.

Thus, if we use our previous example of having increased the **airway radius** (R) by a factor of 5, and thus having reduced the airway resistance by a factor 625, the airflow increases by a proportional value: 625.

Boards Boot Camp High-Yield Compendium

Section 88.0.1   <u>**Mechanical Control of Breathing**</u>

Of course, airway resistance and airflow are not the only determinants to satisfactory respiration. The physical ability to breath is mediated via muscles which, of course, must be functional. Difficulty with breathing, with subsequent insufficient carbon dioxide removal and insufficient oxygen delivery, can be experienced in any disorder that affects the skeletal muscles responsible for the mechanical process of breathing. Such disorders include **ALS**, **advanced myasthenia gravis**, **CVA**, **botulism**, and **tetanus.**

The most important muscle for breathing is the **diaphragm.** The intercostals and accessory respiratory muscles are only used during times of respiratory distress and exercise. Thus, it is the diaphragm that mediates normal breathing at rest. When it contracts, the ribs are lifted upward and outward and the sub-diaphragmatic structures are pushed downward, thereby causing an increase in thoracic size or volume. This increase in volume causes the intrathoracic pressures to change, creating a gradient (pressure difference) between the mouth and the alveoli. In the equation,

Q = ∆P/R (as described previously), we see that a change in the gradient (∆P) causes airflow to increase proportionately. Thus, air enters the lung.

When the diaphragm then relaxes, the abdominal contents are allowed to rise and the ribs are allowed to lower and move inward, causing air to passively be driven out. That is **expiration**.

Therefore, another important means by which to maintain optimal airflow is to maintain a healthy, strong diaphragm since that plays a major role in creating the **pressure gradient** (∆P) that increases airflow. Singers and professional speakers take advantage of this knowledge by developing the diaphragm in order to maximize airflow (optimal inward airflow also allows for optimal outward airflow). The optimized outward airflow during expiration is used to augment the functions and sounds of the larynx.

Another determinant in respiratory success is the level of respiratory system **compliance**. Compliance refers to the distensibility (stretchiness in terms of expandability) of the lung and chest wall. Compliance is inversely proportional to **elastance** (which is determined mostly by the amount of elastic tissue, and refers to the elastic recoil that allows for deflation) and is also inversely proportional to lung and chest wall stiffness.

Patients that have little elastance, such as patients with **alpha-1 antitrypsin deficiency** who have lost much elastin, will therefore have high lung compliance. Patients who have a stiff chest wall, such as patients with **ankylosing spondylitis** or **acute rib fracture,** will also have decreased compliance.

Compliance is described as the amount of volume present for every unit of pressure. Thus, the more volume in the lung at any given time, without a significant increase in pressure, the more the compliance. In other words, the respiratory structures expand to accommodate the increased volume. This can be best calculated as follows:

C = $\Delta V/\Delta P$, where C = compliance, ΔV = change in lung volume, and ΔP equals change in transmural pressure.

Additionally, remember that elastance is the inverse of compliance, as calculated below:

E = 1/C = $\Delta P/\Delta V$, where E = elastance, C = compliance, ΔV = change in lung volume, and ΔP equals change in transmural pressure.

The pressure refers to **transmural pressure** (transpulmonary pressure), the pressure within the alveolus (e.g., "in the lung") minus the **intrapleural pressure** (e.g., the pressure around the lung).

When the diaphragm is contracted, the thoracic cavity enlarges, allowing for a decreased intrapleural pressure that drops to negative values (vacuum-like). So, if pressure is equal to alveolar pressure minus intrapleural pressure, and we give the alveolar pressure an arbitrary value of 0.25 and the intrapleural pressure and arbitrary value of - 5 (NEGATIVE – remember, the chest wall has been expanded), then the transmural pressure would be 0.25 – (-5) = 0.25 + 5 = 5.25. Thus, this would increase transmural pressure. This represents the pressure for lung expansion to occur, and causes air entry and lung filling. The compliance is then determined by how much volume is able to enter for that given pressure. If a tremendous lung volume increase occurs that is significantly larger than the pressure, then the lung is said to be very compliant. However, with this increased transmural pressure that is brought about by the decrease in intrapleural pressure, if only a small volume of air is allowed to enter, then the lung is said to have low compliance.

Emphysema, a type of obstructive lung disease, causes increased lung compliance. This explains why this causes hyperinflated lungs. Conversely, those with **restrictive lung disease** have decreased compliance.

When the diaphragm relaxes after inspiration, that causes the ribs to move inward and downward, effectively causing a significant increase in intrapleural pressure. Thus, pressures within the intrapleural space increase and move to more positive values. This causes a decrease in transpulmonary pressure, which facilitates air exit from the lung.

521

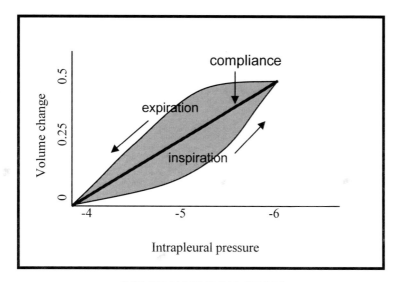

COMPLIANCE DIAGRAM

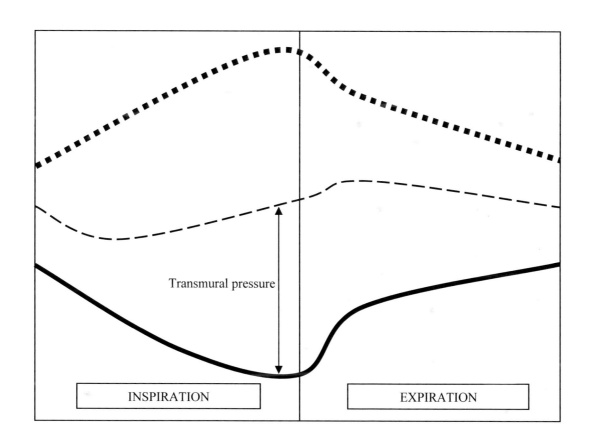

LUNG PRESSURES AND VOLUMES

──── = intrapleural pressure

── ── = alveolar pressure

■ ■ ■ = lung volume

Section 88.0.2 Neurologic Control of Pulmonary Function

Neurologic control of breathing is mediated by the brainstem and cerebral cortex.

The **cerebral cortex** allows a person to voluntarily control their breathing rate, allowing them to voluntarily hyperventilate or hypoventilate. However, the ability to voluntarily hypoventilate is limited by stimulation of peripheral chemoreceptors due to increased serum pCO_2.

The **carotid bodies** and **aortic bodies** contain **peripheral chemoreceptors**.

Generally, the central control centers for respiration are much more sensitive to the effects of increased **pCO_2**, but their response is somewhat delayed. So, although the primary drive comes from the central control centers and is mediated by the effects of rising CO_2, the most immediate and fast response to a sudden increase in serum carbon dioxide (e.g., as experienced with breath-holding) is mediated through the peripheral chemoreceptors.

Despite this effect of CO_2 on peripheral chemoreceptors, the primary role for peripheral chemoreceptors is that of detecting decreasing levels of **oxygen**. Decreased serum oxygen levels cause a strong stimulation of peripheral chemoreceptors. When the carotid bodies are stimulated, they send impulses through afferent nerve fibers that pass through **Hering's nerves** to the **glossopharyngeal nerves**. From there, these impulses are delivered to the **dorsal respiratory area of the medulla**. When the aortic bodies are stimulated, they send afferent impulses through the **vagus nerves** which, in turn, also deliver the impulse to the dorsal respiratory area of the medulla.

The **dorsal respiratory area of the medulla** is all or mostly located within the **nucleus of the tractus solitarius**. The basic rhythm of breathing, via inspiration, originates in this area; this is a spontaneous event that occurs even without incoming stimuli. Breathing rate is increased with input from afferent impulses originating from chemoreceptors. Thus, this area mediates both its rhythmic control as well as rate control via stimulation, via the **phrenic nerves**, to the **diaphragm**.

The **apneustic center**, located in the **lower pons**, stimulates the dorsal respiratory center to produce a large, sustained inspiration. If, through experimentation, it is allowed to function without restraint, it causes the lungs to become almost completely filled and allows only occasional intervening expiratory gasps.

The **pneumotaxic center** is located in the **upper pons**. Its function is to limit inspiration. It mediates this control by sending inhibitory signals to the dorsal respiratory area of the medulla.

The **ventral respiratory group** is located slightly anterior and lateral to the dorsal respiratory area in the medulla, and is found in the **nucleus ambiguus** and the **nucleus retroambiguus**. The neurons of this area are almost completely inactive during normal breathing at rest. However, when the afferent signals coming into the dorsal respiratory area (the area that provides rhythmic inspiratory drive and rate control) become overwhelming, those impulses "spill over" into the ventral respiratory group. The neurons of the ventral respiratory group then contribute to both inspiration and expiration, with greatest effect on the latter via powerful signals it sends to the diaphragm. Thus, it is typically activated during times of stress and exercise.

There are other types of receptors that control breathing. These include:
1) **Lung stretch receptors**
   - These are located in the smooth muscle of the airways and are stimulated by lung distention; when stimulated, they cause a reflex decrease in respiration rate known as the **Hering-Breuer reflex**.
2) **Joint and muscle receptors**
   - These play a role in increasing respiration rate during exercise.
3) **Irritant receptors**
   - These are found between epithelial cells that line the airways; they detect irritating substances and produce an afferent signal that is carried through the vagus nerve to the medulla. The result is a rapid inspiration of air, then closing of the epiglottis, then forceful contraction of abdominal muscles and intercostals. Finally, the epiglottis opens suddenly, allowing the air in the lung to explode out in the form of a **cough**. This is the cough reflex.
4) **J receptors**
   - These are also known as juxtacapillary receptors, and are situated next to ("juxta") capillaries on the alveoli; engorgement of the capillaries, such as what occurs with "back up" of blood secondary to CHF, causes activation of these J receptors. Their activation results in shallow, fast breathing.

Certain pathologic breathing patterns can be established, depending upon the stimulus presented.

For instance, there is **Cheyne-Stokes respiration**. It is characterized by a waxing and waning in amplitude (volume of air inspired). In other words, each inspiration gets progressively deeper, then reaches a peak, then gets progressively shallower; the cycle repeats itself continuously. It is actually caused by recurrent, cyclic episodes of apnea; the apnea causes hypercapnea (increased CO2 levels), which then cause deeper breathing. As the carbon dioxide is blown off, the depth of inspirations decreases. Then, another apneic episode occurs, and the whole process repeats itself. It is seen in severe congestive heart failure or arrhythmias (because of poor perfusion), central sleep apnea, and a variety of neurologic diseases resulting from head injury, stroke, or brain tumors of any of the respiratory centers in the brainstem.

Kussmaul breathing, on the other hand, is very deep and, often, rapid, and occurs to compensate for extreme cases of metabolic acidosis (such as with diabetic ketoacidosis [DKA]).

Biot breathing, also known as ataxic respiration, features periods of quick, shallow breathing followed by periods of apnea. It results from damage to the medulla, and is seen as a consequence to, among many things, trauma or cerebrovascular accident to that area.

Section 88.0.3   <u>Pulmonary Circulation</u>

When **alveolar oxygen concentration** drops, the blood vessels nearby constrict; this is opposite of what happens in normal systemic vasculature. This mechanism in pulmonary vasculature assures that blood is shunted towards those parts of the lung that are better oxygenated.

In any case, the **blood pressures** overall are much lower in the pulmonary circulation than what they are in the systemic circulation. Generally, pulmonary arterial pressure is normally about 15% of aortic pressure.

In addition, **pulmonary vascular resistance** is much lower in the pulmonary circulatory system, ensuring optimal blood flow through the lung structures. Pulmonary perfusion is driven by the right ventricle.

When a patient is upright, the perfusion of the lung is different in different zones of the lung. The apex (tip) of the lung is considered **zone one**; zone one has the lowest blood flow. This is because the alveolar pressures in zone 1 are the highest, and can be even higher than pulmonary arterial pressure, minimizing the amount of blood flow to that area.

In **zone 2**, arterial pressure of the lung generally exceeds that of alveoli; this is because of gravitational effect on the blood.

In **zone 3**, the lowest part of the lung, gravitational effect is greatest on the vasculature, and causes both arterial and venous pulmonary pressures to exceed alveolar pressures. Thus, blood flow is the highest in zone 3.

However, the effects on alveoli by the arterial and venous pressures play a role in ventilation. Because of the inherent structure of the lung itself, ventilation (gas exchange) is the lowest in zone 1 and, because bronchi drive inspired air down, greatest in zone 3. However, the low ventilation in zone 1 is NOT proportional to the decreased blood flow in zone one; instead, there is far more ventilation that occurs in zone 1 as compared to blood flow in zone 1. Thus, in zone one, ventilation (though the lowest in the lung) far exceeds blood flow (which is even lower). Therefore, the **V/Q ratio** (comparison of ventilation to blood flow) is the highest in zone 1 of lung. Conversely, although ventilation occurs the most in zone 3 and blood flow occurs the most in zone 3, the amount of blood flow in zone 3 far exceeds the amount of ventilation. Thus, the V/Q ratio is the lowest in zone 3 of the lung.

Normal V/Q ratios of the lung can be changed by a variety of pathologies; any change is termed a "**V/Q defect**" or "**V/Q mismatch**.". With **pulmonary embolism (PE)**, there is an obstruction to blood flow in the pulmonary arterial system. The result is that ventilation remains the same while blood flow decreases (because of the

525

obstruction). Thus, V is the same and Q decreases, causing the V/Q to increase. On the other hand, if there is obstruction of an airway, ventilation will be significantly decreased while blood flow remains the same (or slightly decreases secondary to hypoxia). Accordingly, the V/Q is decreased because of the huge decrease in V (ventilation). When V/Q equals 0 (e.g., there is no ventilation), that is termed a **shunt**.

Section 88.0.4   <u>**Pulmonary Edema**</u>

There are 2 major causes for pulmonary edema (fluid accumulation in the lung):
    1) left-sided heart failure (CHF)
    2) damage to pulmonary capillary membranes (e.g., ARDS)

In both cases, water leaves the vascular space of pulmonary capillaries and enters lung structures.

Section 88.1   <u>**LUNG VOLUMES**</u>

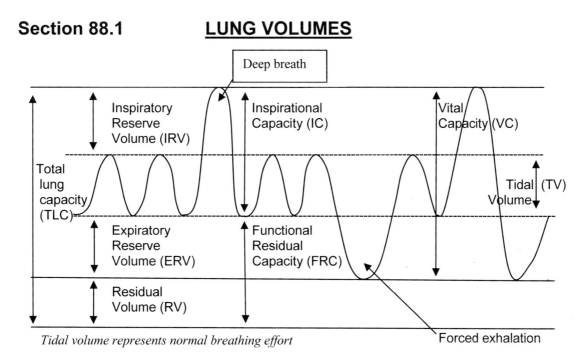

Tidal volume represents normal breathing effort

Lung Disease & Lung Volumes

	Obstructive	**Restrictive**
Vital capacity	0 or decreased	**DECREASED**
Functional Residual Capacity	increased	decreased
Residual Volume	**INCREASED**	DECREASED
Total Lung Capacity	INCREASED	DECREASED

Notes:

Section 89.0   FRANK-STARLING LAW

Frank-Starling Law states that when increased quantities of blood flow into the heart (resulting in increased preload), this stretches the walls of the heart chambers. As a result of the stretch, the cardiac muscle contracts with increased force and, within limits, with increased cardiac output.

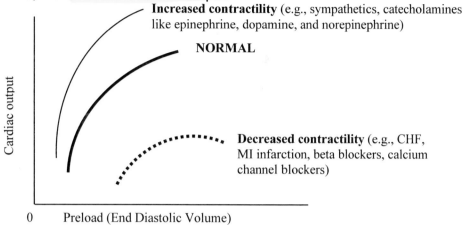

Increased contractility (e.g., sympathetics, catecholamines like epinephrine, dopamine, and norepinephrine)

NORMAL

Decreased contractility (e.g., CHF, MI infarction, beta blockers, calcium channel blockers)

Section 89.1   ELECTRICAL PATHWAY OF HEART

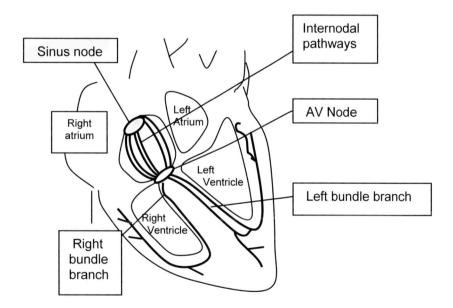

Cardiac muscle is a syncytium; this is made possible by way of intercalated discs. The syncytial nature of the heart allows the stimulation to spread directly from cell to cell. Such spread is prevented between the cells of the atria and ventricles as all conduction from the atria to the ventricles has to pass through the AV node.

Section 89.1.0   <u>**Cardiac Action Potential**</u>

<u>Ventricles, Atria, and Purkinje fibers</u>
- The ventricles, atria, and Purkinje system (left and right bundles) have long-duration action potentials; this is especially magnified in the Purkinje fibers.
- Their resting membrane potentials are stable (at about -90 mV)

<u>Sinoatrial node (SA node)</u>
- The sinoatrial node is the pacemaker of the heart, and so exhibits automaticity
- It has an unstable resting membrane potential
- When the SA node fires too slowly, the AV node will demonstrate "latent automaticity," providing the rhythmic impulse that drives heart contraction. If the AV node fires too slowly, the His-Purkinje system will demonstrate automaticity, thereby generating the impulse for a heartbeat.

<u>ACTION POTENTIAL: Ventricles, Atria, and Purkinje fibers</u>

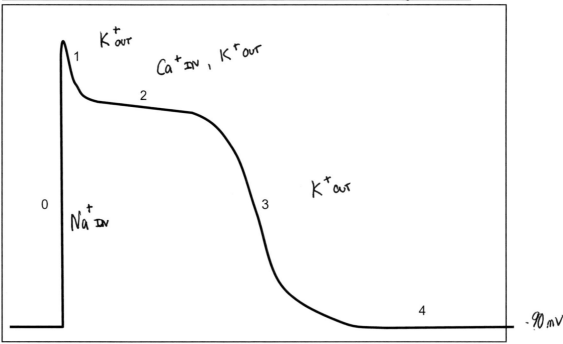

The 5 phases of the cardiac action potential for ventricles, atria, and Purkinje fibers are demonstrated.

Boards Boot Camp High-Yield Compendium

Phase 0
- Is the upstroke
- Is caused by sodium entry into the cell that causes depolarization of the cell

Phase 1
- Represents a short moment of repolarization
- Is caused by mostly by potassium moving out of the cell, along with a decrease in sodium entry

Phase 2
- Is the plateau
- Is caused by calcium entry into the cell, along with continued potassium exit

Phase 3
- Is repolarization
- Is due to the predominant exit of potassium from the cell

Phase 4
- Is the resting membrane potential
- Is due to an equal amount of inward and outward current (movement of ions) -90mV

PACEMAKER

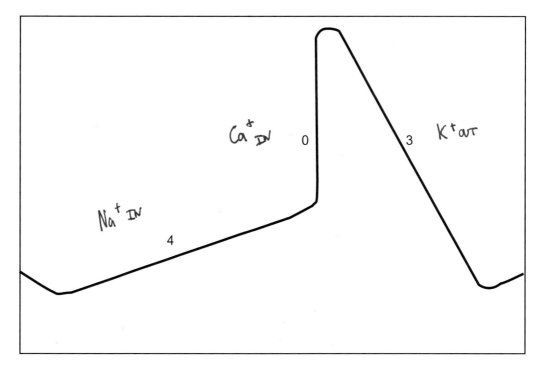

The 3 phases of the cardiac action potential for the sinoatrial node (SA node) are demonstrated.

Phase 0
- Is the <u>upstroke</u>
- Is caused by calcium entry into the cell that causes the final depolarization of the cell

Phase 3
- Is the <u>repolarization</u>
- Is caused by potassium departure from the cell

Phase 4
- Is the <u>slow depolarization</u> of the cell
- Is responsible for the automaticity of the SA node
- Is caused by slow sodium entry into the cell

Section 89.2   <u>Physiology of Cardiac Arrhythmias</u>

In order to appreciate cardiac arrhythmias, it is important to understand what each part of an EKG represents:

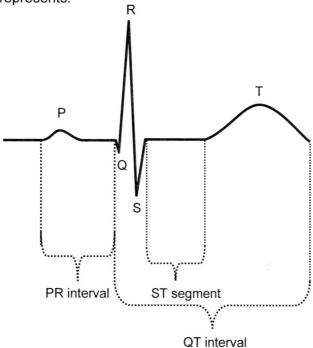

P wave
- Is depolarization of the atria Na^+ IN

Q wave
- Is the start to the depolarization of the ventricles Na^+ IN

QRS complex
- Is depolarization of the ventricles right before contraction
- Repolarization of the atria occurs at the same time, but cannot be visualized because it is obscured by the QRS complex

T wave
- Represents ventricular repolarization K^+ exit

PR interval

- Is the period of time in which the impulse is conducted through the AV node
- Is lengthened during AV block (heart block), a situation in which the impulse is slowed pathologically through the AV node, delaying the conduction from the atria to the ventricles
- Is decreased during activation by the sympathetic nervous system, thereby decreasing the amount of time it takes for the impulse to get from the atria to the ventricles

ST segment

- Is continued ventricular depolarization during ventricular contraction during which all parts of the ventricle have become depolarized
- Generally, will usually become elevated with damaging pathology (injury) occurring at the heart's surface, in the leads representing that part of the heart
- Generally, will usually become depressed with ischemia or infarction not occurring at the heart's surface, in the leads representing that part of the heart

Surface sees 1st blood so when ischemia its a unstable MI

QT interval

- Is the entire period of time during which the ventricles are depolarized and then repolarized
- Represents that period of time of ventricular contraction

Section 89.2.1 SINUS RHYTHM ANOMALIES

Abnormal sinus rhythms = abnormal rhythms generated by the sinus node (SA node)

Stimulation of the SA node → tachycardia (heart rate > 100 bpm)
Etiologies: 1) increased body temperature
2) sympathetic stimulation (via beta one receptor activation by way of direct neuronal stimulation (such as T2, T3, etc.) or by way of epinephrine stimulation delivered by the blood)
3) toxicities (e.g., digitalis overdose)

Inhibition of the SA node → bradycardia (heart rate < 60 bpm)
    Etiologies: 1) parasympathetic stimulation (via the vagus nerve)

Section 89.2.2   AV BLOCK

AV block is a block at the atrioventricular node that stops impulses that arose from the SA node, blocking those impulses from being transmitted to the ventricles.

    Etiologies:
    1) ischemia of the AV node or bundle
    2) compression of the AV node or bundle by scarred tissue
           or calcifications
    3) inflammation of the AV node or bundle, occurring most
           likely secondary to acute rheumatic fever, – Ⓒ heart
           myocarditis, or diphtheria ε2 dangahn, grey throat
    4) hyperparasympathetic stimulation via the vagus

The types of AV block are:
    A)   first degree heart block = PR interval of > 0.20 seconds (more
           than 5 small squares on EKG)
    B)   second degree heart block
    C)   third degree heart block – the atria and ventricles operate
           independently. When this comes and goes, it is known as Stoke-
           Adams syndrome.

Section 89.2.3   PREMATURE CONTRACTIONS

Premature contractions = extrasystoles

Premature contractions are caused by ectopic foci that generate independent cardiac impulses, thereby creating extra contractions.

Etiologies if ectopic foci:
    1)   local ischemia
    2)   compression of cardiac tissue by pressure generated by an
            atherosclerotic plaque
    3)   toxicity caused by nicotine, caffeine, or other drugs

Ectopic foci can originate in the atria, the AV junction, or the ventricle. Those that originate in the atria cause premature atria contractions (PACs). Those that originate in the AV junction cause premature contractions with the P wave superimposed on the QRS, and therefore the P wave is not visible. Ectopic foci in the ventricles create premature ventricular contractions (PVCs), creating a prolonged, wide QRS because the ectopic foci impulse must travel through muscle the entire way instead of through the Purkinje system which is the normal route and a much faster system.

Section 89.2.4   PAROXYSMAL TACHYCARDIA

These tachycardias are considered to be caused by re-entrant pathways that allow impulses to "loop back," causing the same tissue to be rapidly self re-excited. Since this is so rapid, this impulse and the resulting muscle contraction exceeds the internal pacemaker speed of the heart; hence, this process becomes the new pacemaker of the heart. Paroxysmal tachycardia means that the rapid heart rate occurs spontaneously and in bursts, returning to normal within seconds, minutes, or days. Typically these are treated with quinidine or lidocaine since these two drugs block sodium channels in the cardiac tissue and, consequently, inhibit the impulse generating the tachycardia. There is atrial paroxysmal tachycardia and ventricular paroxysmal tachycardia. If the tachycardia is generated by the sinus node, it is considered to be sinus tachycardia (which is discussed in an earlier section). However, if the tachycardia is caused by any site in the atrium other than the sinus node (sinoatrial node), it is considered a type of atrial paroxysmal tachycardia. It will generate an inverted P wave because of atrial depolarization moving in the opposite direction as normal. When the tachycardia is generated from the AV node, P waves may be obscured or inverted; this type of tachycardia is known as supraventricular tachycardia (SVT).

Ventricular paroxysmal tachycardia is much rarer than the aforementioned conditions. When it does occur, it typically results from significant ischemic damage to the ventricle and frequently, subsequently, causes life-threatening ventricular fibrillation.

[handwritten margin note: Type I antiarrhythmic]

Section 89.2.5   <u>VENTRICULAR FIBRILLATION</u>

This is the most serious of the cardiac arrhythmias. Multiple impulses are generated in various parts of the ventricular muscle, causing the ventricles to have multiple areas contracting at the same time while other portions are relaxed. Consequently, there is little to no cardiac output because of the lack of coordination of contraction and the speed of the contractions that are occurring. The movement of impulses "around" the heart is termed "circus movement."

Under normal conditions, when an impulse moves through the ventricle, that single impulse eventually ends because, as depolarization occurs, the skeletal muscle then becomes refractory to any further stimulation for a while. However, circus movement with the never ending movement of an impulse from one part of the ventricle to another is possible because of 3 conditions:

1) shortened refractory period in muscle which may be generated by repetitive electrical stimulation or by epinephrine administration

2) increased distance between impulses; for instance, once the impulse is generated and moves around the heart, by the time it reaches its original location, that location may already have recovered from its refractory state and be ready for another depolarizing event. This possibility is increased if the heart itself is increased in size, thereby increasing the distance that the impulse must travel before returning to its original site. Hence, dilated hearts or enlarged hearts are more prone to this.

3) decreased speed (velocity) of impulse conduction; again, if the impulse itself travels very slowly, the likelihood of the heart issue to have recovered from its refractory state prior to return of that impulse is much greater. Impulses will travel slowly during cardiac ischemia and during hyperkalemia.

The purpose of defibrillation is to make all parts of the heart refractory to further stimulation (for only a brief period of time!), thus giving the heart the opportunity to reset itself with normal single impulses without circus impulse generation and movement.

Section 89.2.6   **ATRIAL FIBRILLATION**

The process and causes of atrial fibrillation are the same as those for ventricular fibrillation, except that they occur in the atria. And, of course, enlarged atria increase the likelihood of such an occurrence; valvular disease is a frequent cause for that enlargement. As with the ventricles, if there is atrial fibrillation, the atria do not pump blood. Consequently, without functional atrial pumping, the ventricles receive much less blood, decreasing ventricular efficiency by 20-30%.

Atrial flutter is different than AFib. Atrial flutter is caused by a single large impulse wave that travels round and round in the atria. Consequently, when one atrium is contracted the other one is relaxed, and vice versa.

Section 89.2.7   EKGs

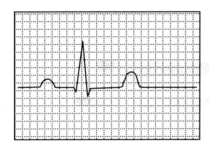

Normal EKG

1st Degree AV Block
(PR interval > 5 blocks)

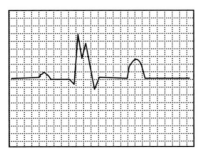

Bundle Branch Block
(if in V5 and V6 = left bundle branch block; if in V1 and V2 = right bundle branch block)

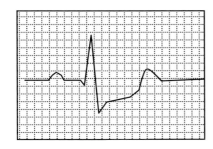

ST segment depression

Sparing myocardial surface

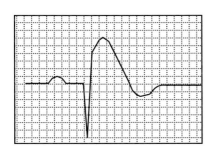

ST segment elevation
(with T wave inversion)

Surface involved

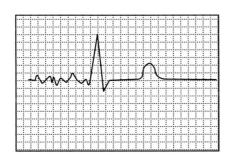

Atrial fibrillation

"√"

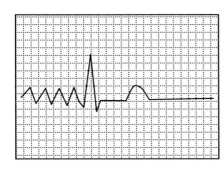

Atrial flutter

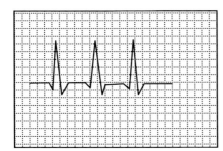

Supraventricular Tachycardia

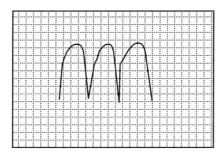

Ventricular Tachycardia

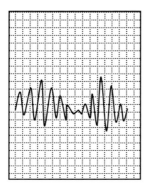

Torsade de Pointe
(note that it seems to "wind" around the
same baseline)

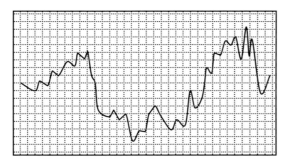

Ventricular Fibrillation
(note the erratic rapid pattern
with NO discernable baseline)

Section 89.3   <u>CARDIOVASCULAR FACTS TO KNOW</u>

1. **Pulmonary vasculature pressures** are much smaller than systemic vascular pressures; e.g. typical pulmonary blood pressure is 25/8, with mean arterial pressure (MAP) = 16. **Mean pulmonary wedge pressure** (the pressure at the pulmonary capillaries) is 8 mm Hg.

2. **Pulse pressure** = systolic pressure – diastolic pressure

3. Most blood at any given time is in the venous system.

4. **Speed (velocity) of the blood flow** is inversely proportional to the total cross-sectional area of the blood vessels through which it is traveling. Accordingly, blood flows the slowest through the capillaries since they, cumulatively, have the greatest total cross-sectional area. The aorta conducts the blood with the greatest velocity.   ↑ resistance

5. Individual vessel diameter plays a major role in **resistance to blood flow**; this is determined by Poiseuille's Law. According to the law, vascular resistance is directly proportional to blood viscosity, directly proportional to the length of the blood vessel, and inversely proportional to the radius of the blood vessel (to the 4th power! – hence, blood vessel diameter is an extremely potent aspect of determining vascular resistance).

    For example, if the radius of a blood vessel doubles (e.g., two times its normal size), resistance will change by the inverse of radius x 2 (because of doubled diameter) to the 4th power. Therefore, resistance will be inverse of 16, which means that resistance will be 1/16th of what it was to begin with. What this means is that blood flow will be 16 times greater than what it was before the blood vessel dilated to twice its diameter!

6. **Conductance** is the ease with which blood flows through a blood vessel and is determined by 1/resistance (the inverse of resistance) – using the aforementioned example where resistance is 1/16th of what it was, conductance will be 16 times what it was.

7. **Compliance = capacitance** = the total amount of blood that can remain or be stores in a particular blood vessel at a given pressure = increase in volume divided by increase in pressure = distensibility x volume...in other words, the greater the compliance of a blood vessel, the more easily it is able to distend at any given pressure.

8. **Veins** have generally about 24 times greater compliance that arteries of the same size.

9. Sympathetic stimulation of blood vessels (except in skeletal and cardiac muscle) decreases the compliance of those blood vessels and incurs vasoconstriction, with the latter thereby also increasing resistance.

10. The 2 most important elements to affect pulse pressure are **stroke volume** (the amount of blood pumped into the aorta with each heartbeat) and arterial compliance. For example, when stroke volume is increased, pulse pressure is increased.

11. **Aortic valve stenosis** decreases blood flow with each heartbeat, therefore little blood or pressure is generated during systole; hence, it decreases pulse pressure.

12. **Patent ductus arteriosus** results in some blood that was pumped into the aorta being distributed to the pulmonary artery during diastole. This significantly decreases the diastolic pressure, thereby significantly increasing the pulse pressure.

13. **Aortic regurgitation** allows blood that was pumped into the aorta during systole to flow back into the heart during diastole (when the valve is normally supposed to be closed – which it is not in this condition). This decreases diastolic pressure and, therefore, increases pulse pressure.

14. The average overall body-wide pressure in blood vessels during one cardiac cycle = the perfusion pressure presented to organs = Mean blood pressure = **Mean arterial pressure** = MAP

15. **MAP = $P_{diastolic}$ + 1/3 ($P_{systolic}$ − $P_{diastolic}$)**

    = $P_{diastolic}$ + 1/3 (Pulse Pressure)

    = 2/3 diastolic pressure + 1/3 systolic pressure

    = (CO x SVR) + CVP

    = approximately (CO x SVR),
    where $P_{diastolic}$ = diastolic blood pressure, $P_{systolic}$ = systolic blood pressure, CO = cardiac output, SVR = systemic vascular resistance, and CVR = central venous pressure (which can usually be omitted due to its typical negligible value, allowing for a close approximation of MAP to be easily calculated)

16. The average MAP for a young healthy adult is about 93.3.

17. **Normal MAP = 70-110 mm Hg**; MAPs less than that put organs at risk of receiving inadequate perfusion and, thus, at risk of suffering ischemia

18. The **valves in the veins** are positioned normally to only allow blood flow to move towards the heart. The major stimulator for venous movement is actually the contraction of skeletal muscle in which the veins are located. The combination of surrounding skeletal muscle contraction along with valves preventing backward flow during skeletal muscle relaxation is known as the "venous pump" or "muscle pump".

19.   Failure of venous valves causes **varicose veins**. Because of the venous blood stasis, persons can suffer from edema of the feet and legs when standing.

20.   Four forces determine **fluid filtration through capillaries**:

1)   capillary hydrostatic pressure (water pressure which forces fluid outward through the capillary wall)
2)   interstitial hydrostatic pressure (water pressure which forces fluid inward through the capillary wall)
3)   plasma oncotic (colloid osmotic) pressure (which draws water, via osmosis, into capillaries)
4)   interstitial oncotic (colloid osmotic) pressure (which draws water, via osmosis, into interstitial spaces)

These 4 forces work together, with the greatest force directing the ultimate (net) direction of fluid flow across the capillary walls.

21.   Most **oncotic** pressure is generated by the plasma protein known as albumin. Albumin has a negative charge, so besides having a draw simply because of its charge it also attracts Na which has a positive charge; Na binds to it, attracting water its way, as well.

22.   With each cardiac contraction, the left ventricle pumps out a portion or fraction of the blood in it; this is known as **ejection fraction** (EF). EF = (stroke volume/end-diastolic volume) x 100% (normal range = 55-80%)

23.   The **cardiac cycle** is the entire cycle of heart filling and pumping:

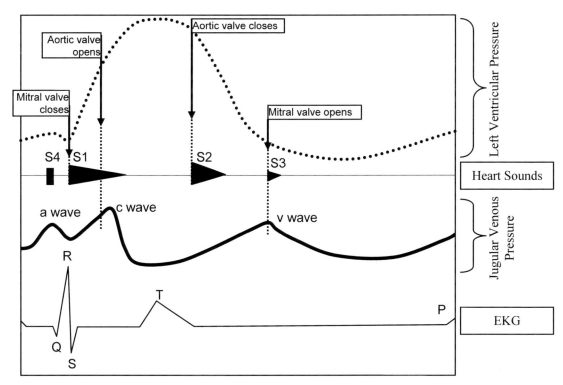

a wave = atrial contraction; c wave = right ventricular contraction;
v wave = increasing atrial pressure due to closed tricuspid valve

24.   **Cardiac output** is the volume of blood pumped by the heart in 1 minute.

25.   **Cardiac output = CO = stroke volume x heart rate**
       = [EDV-ESV] x heart rate, where EDV = end-diastolic volume and ESV = end-systolic volume.

26.   Stroke volume is the volume of blood pumped by the blood with one
       contraction. **Stroke volume = SV = end-diastolic volume – end-systolic
       volume**

27.   **Average resting cardiac output** is 5.6 L/min for a male, and 4.9 L/min for a
       female.

28.   **Heart failure** is characterized by inadequate cardiac output. Its diagnosis is
       confirmed by echocardiogram, wherein ejection fraction is measured. A low
       ejection fraction is diagnostic for heart failure.

29.   Most cases of **high cardiac output** are due to decreased total peripheral resistance. Prolonged high cardiac output can cause heart failure due to taxing the heart too much. Chronic conditions associated with high cardiac output (and that can, therefore, lead to high output cardiac failure) are:

       1) **Beriberi** – due to thiamine deficiency.
       2) **Anemia** – this causes a decrease in oxygen delivery to tissues, resulting in vasodilatation; it also causes a decrease in blood viscosity (due to decreased RBC numbers), increasing the cardiac output.
       3) **Hyperthyroidism** – hyperthyroidism increases metabolic demand for oxygen in all tissues, resulting in a reflex vasodilatation to supply more oxygen.
       4) **Arteriovenous shunt** – without the capillary connection between the arterial and venous system, there is significant decrease in peripheral resistance.

30.   Systemic vascular resistance is the resistance to blood flow in blood vessels that must be overcome in order to have blood flow.
Systemic vascular resistance
= SVR
= total peripheral resistance
= TPR
= MAP/CO
= mean arterial pressure/cardiac output

Section 89.4.0   <u>Skeletal Muscle Blood Vessels</u>

During exercise, vasodilatation occurs secondary to:
     Beta-two receptor activation
     Potassium ion elevation in blood, locally
     Hydrogen ion elevation in blood, locally
     Lactic acid elevation
     Carbon dioxide elevation
     Adenosine elevation, locally

Vasodilatation becomes quite pronounced with significant sympathetic stimulation (via beta–two receptors).

Section 89.4.1 Cardiac Muscle Blood Vessels
(a.k.a. Coronary Arteries)

Vasodilatory causes include:
  Potassium ion elevation in blood, locally
  Hydrogen ion elevation in blood, locally
  Carbon dioxide elevation
  Bradykinin elevation
  Prostaglandin elevation
  Adenosine elevation, locally
  Beta-two receptor activation

While sympathetic activation promotes coronary artery vasodilation, local effects like some of those noted above have, comparatively, the most potent effects.

Section 90.0   HEMOGLOBIN SATURATION CURVES

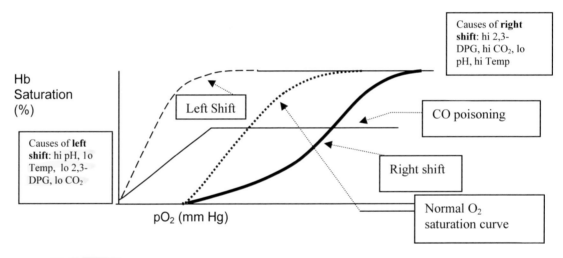

A left-shift causes the hemoglobin to be more saturated at the same oxygen concentration; this means that the hemoglobin in a left-shift is less likely to release its oxygen to tissues. Conversely, right-shift of hemoglobin saturation means that the hemoglobin is less saturated at the same oxygen concentration; thus, hemoglobin undergoing right-shift saturation more easily and readily releases its oxygen to tissues.

Causes of a right shift are high 2,3-DPG, elevated serum carbon dioxide concentrations, decreased serum pH, or elevated body temperatures. 2,3-DPG is a by-product of metabolism; increased levels generally reflect increased metabolic rate. Thus, the oxygen demands are met during this increased metabolic rate because oxygen is more readily released by hemoglobin. Increased metabolic rates also cause an increase in carbon dioxide production from tissues; that carbon dioxide will also increase the likelihood for hemoglobin release of oxygen. Carbon dioxide levels can also rise secondary to respiratory compromise. Due to the respiratory compromise, oxygenation of the blood will not be optimal, but release to tissues of whatever

Boards Boot Camp High-Yield Compendium

oxygen is gained will be optimized to maintain homeostasis as best as possible. High metabolic rates can reduce serum pH; one mechanism for this is via the excess production of lactic acid. Thus, such acidic conditions that may result from increased metabolic activity will also facilitate hemoglobin's release of oxygen to tissues. Lastly, an increase in body temperature will encourage easier release of oxygen from hemoglobin; increased body temperature can be a result of increased metabolism. Thus, the improved availability of oxygen to tissues can help to meet these increased metabolic demands.

Section 90.0.1   <u>TYPES OF HEMOGLOBIN</u>

Normal Adult Hb = HbA ($\alpha_2\beta_2$) & HbA$_2$ ($\alpha_2\delta_2$)
Fetal Hb = HbF ($\alpha_2\gamma_2$)   *NOTE: Oxygen affinity of HbF is similar to left shift of adult Hb*
Embryonic Hb = Gower 1 ($\zeta_2\varepsilon_2$)

Myoglobin (in red skeletal muscle) is similar to hemoglobin, but its oxygen affinity is similar to left shift of adult Hb

Sickle cell anemia features HbS ($\alpha_2\beta^s_2$)
Alpha-thalassemia features Hb Bart (γ_4) and HbH (β_4)
Beta-thalassemia features HbF and HbA$_2$

Section 91.0   <u>RENAL TRANSPORT</u>

REMEMBER!!! The kidney does more than filter blood and handle electrolytes. It also converts vitamin D to its active form, produces erythropoietin, and produces renin in response to low Na delivery to macula densa in DCT (distal convoluted tubule) and/or low blood pressure in glomerulus (as detected by juxtaglomerular cells).

Proximal Convoluted Tubule

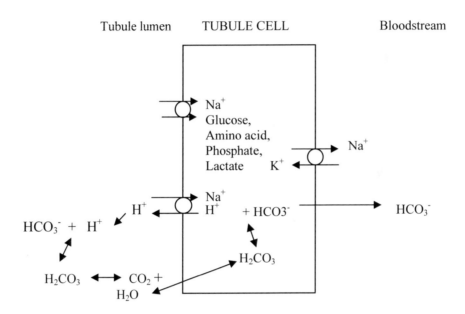

Tubule lumen   TUBULE CELL   Bloodstream

Na$^+$
Glucose,
Amino acid,
Phosphate,   Na$^+$
Lactate   K$^+$

Na$^+$
H$^+$ H$^+$ + HCO3$^-$ HCO$_3^-$

HCO$_3^-$ + H$^+$ H$_2$CO$_3$

H$_2$CO$_3$ CO$_2$ +   H$_2$O

Thick Ascending Loop of Henle

Tubule lumen   TUBULE CELL   bloodstream

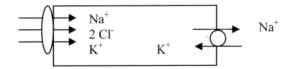

Na$^+$ Na$^+$
2 Cl$^-$
K$^+$ K$^+$

Boards Boot Camp High-Yield Compendium

(early) Distal Convoluted Tubule

Tubule lumen   TUBULE CELL   bloodstream

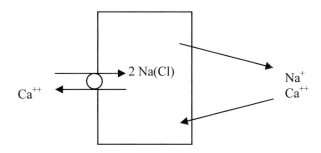

(late) Distal Convoluted Tubule/Collecting Duct

Tubule lumen   TUBULE CELL   bloodstream

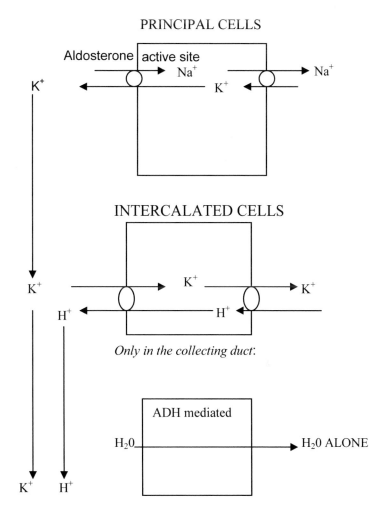

Boards Boot Camp High-Yield Compendium

Section 91.2   <u>RENAL FACTS</u>

Glomerular filtration = filtration of fluid from glomerular capillaries into the renal tubules.

Renal reabsorption = the process of reabsorbing substances from the renal tubules into the peritubular capillaries.

Renal or Tubular Secretion = process of secreting water and solutes into the renal tubules for excretion.

Urinary Excretion = loss of substances via urine.

Nephron = the tuft of glomerular capillaries + the glomerulus + Bowman's capsule + the renal tubule.

The **proximal convoluted tubule (PCT)** is located in the outer area of the kidney known as the cortex.

The **Loop of Henle** dips into the deep parts of the kidney known as the medulla.

The **distal convoluted tubule (DCT)** lies in the cortex (outer part) of the kidney.

The **collecting duct** starts in the cortex of the kidney and descends into the medulla.

Renal blood flow constitutes, on average, 22% of the cardiac output. Blood enters the renal artery, then branches to smaller blood vessels, eventually reaching the afferent arterioles. The glomerular capillaries are branches of the afferent arterioles. After the glomerular capillaries pass through the glomerulus, they coalesce to form the efferent arterioles. The efferent arterioles lead to another capillary network known as the peritubular capillaries. These surround the tubules. There are also specialized peritubular capillaries known as the vasa recta that dip into the renal medulla while running parallel to the loop of Henle. The peritubular capillaries progressively coalesce, forming ever larger venous structures, and finally empty into the renal vein. Hence, the kidneys have two distinct sets of capillaries beds: the glomerular capillaries and the peritubular capillaries.

Renal clearance measures the kidney's excretion abilities (e.g., ability to completely remove something from the body). Clearance is a function of glomerular filtration + secretion of substances from the peritubular capillaries to renal tubules + reabsorption actions of the renal tubule of molecules back into the body. Technically, renal clearance is defined as the net volume of a substance removed from the blood by the kidneys and excreted into the urine.

Renal Clearance = $(U \times V)/P_A$, where U = solute concentration in urine, V = volume of urine produced per minute, and P_A = solute concentration in plasma (mg/100 mL plasma). In other words, the higher the urine concentration of the solute being measured, the more of it is being cleared from the body (e.g., excreted via urine), making the renal clearance higher.

Boards Boot Camp High-Yield Compendium

Renal plasma flow = the amount of plasma (blood minus cells) reaching the kidneys per unit of time = **RPF = renal clearance/extraction ratio**.

Extraction ratio is the ratio of solute that has entered the kidneys and has successfully been excreted in the urine. An extraction ratio of 0.5 would mean that half of the solute was excreted, whereas an extraction ratio of 1 would mean that all of it was excreted. **Para-aminohippurate (PAH)** has an excretion ratio of nearly 1, meaning that nearly all of the PAH presented to the kidney is excreted out into the urine. Thus, PAH is typically used in PAH clearance determinations, as it makes determining RPF (renal plasma flow) easier.
If PAH is used, then RPF = renal clearance/1 = renal clearance.
So, if renal clearance can be determined for PAH (via the calculation $[UxV]/P_A$), then renal plasma flow can be inferred from that since, with PAH, renal clearance = renal plasma flow.

Renal blood flow is the volume of whole blood, including cellular constituents, delivered to the kidney during a period of time.
Renal blood flow = RBF = RPF x (1/1-Hct), where RPF = renal plasma flow and Hct = hematocrit).

Section 91.3   <u>GLOMERULAR FILTRATION RATE</u>

Glomerular filtration rate (GFR) is affected by many things:

- decreased GFR is associated with decreased glomerular capillary filtration coefficient (such as situations in which the glomerular capillary membrane (endothelium) is thickened, e.g. chronic hypertension and diabetes mellitus)

- decreased by increased Bowman's capsule pressures, such as those encountered by urinary tract obstruction

- decreased by increased glomerular capillary oncotic pressure

- increased by increased glomerular capillary hydrostatic pressure, such as that found with hypertension (although this effect is frequently buffered by "auto regulation" which somewhat minimizes the effect of blood pressure on glomerular capillaries)

- decreased by decreased glomerular capillary hydrostatic pressure, such as that found with dilated efferent arterioles (like what is found with ACE inhibitors)

- decreased by sympathetic stimulation because it stimulates constriction of both the afferent and efferent arterioles

- increased by angiotensin II because, although angiotensin II constricts both the afferent and efferent arterioles, it constricts the efferents more, thereby increasing glomerular capillary hydrostatic pressures.

-This can all be expressed as:

$$GFR = K_f [(P_{cap}-P_{BS})-(\pi_{cap}-\pi_{BS})],$$

where P_{cap} = hydrostatic (water) pressure in glomerular capillaries, P_{BS} = hydrostatic pressure in Bowman's space, π_{cap} = capillary oncotic pressure, and π_{BS} = Bowman's space oncotic pressure.

So, P_{cap} increases with afferent arteriole vasodilation or efferent arteriole constriction. P_{BS} increases with urolithiasis. π_{cap} decreases with liver failure.

Section 91.4   Proximal Convoluted Tubule Function

* about 65% of the water, Na, Cl, K, and other electrolytes that are presented to the PCT are reabsorbed at the PCT
* amino acids are reabsorbed at the PCT

Section 91.5   Loop of Henle Function

* the descending thin segment dips into the medulla
* the descending thin segment is highly permeable to water, allowing much of the water therein to be reabsorbed into the hypertonic peritubular interstitium; therefore, this part of the tubule plays an important role in concentrating urine
* the ascending thin and ascending thick segments are virtually impermeable to water, but large amounts of Na, K, and Cl are reabsorbed at this point (via the co-transporter that transports 1 Na, 2 Cl, and 1 K as a unit – this is most active in the thick ascending segment)

Section 91.6   Distal Convoluted Tubule and Collecting Duct Function

* the <u>early</u> distal convoluted tubule (DCT) forms part of the juxtaglomerular complex; it also is impermeable to water and urea. Na and Cl are reabsorbed in this area. *exchanged for Ca*
* the <u>late</u> DCT and collecting tubule function similarly because they contain the same cell types as one another:
    1) principal cells – absorb Na and water and exchange the Na for K, such that Na is removed from the lumen and the K is added to the lumen; this activity is controlled by aldosterone
    2) intercalated cells – absorb K ions and secrete, in exchange, hydrogen ions to the tubule lumen
* the <u>late</u> DCT and collecting tubule are virtually impermeable to urea

551

*   the collecting tubule in the renal medulla has variable water permeability: it becomes highly permeable to water, allowing water reabsorption in the presence of antidiuretic hormone (ADH); without ADH, it is impermeable to water.

Section 92.0   <u>Modulators of Fluid and Blood Pressure Maintenance</u>

1.   ADH (anti-diuretic hormone)
2.   SNS (sympathetic nervous system)
3.   Renin (and angiotensin, aldosterone)
4. H_2O ingestion (stimulated by hypothalamus via "thirst")
PLUS other more minor contributors: ANP, NO

atria sketch

Section 93.0   <u>FLUIDS FACTS</u>

The total amount of body water averages about 60% of body weight.

Total body water = intracellular fluid (2/3 of total) + extracellular fluid (1/3 of total)

Extracellular fluid = interstitial fluid (3/4 of total) + plasma (1/4 of total)

Plasma comprises 60% of blood; the other 40% is comprised of RBCs (the latter is the hematocrit).

The pH of the plasma should be 7.35-7.45. Deviations from normal pH indicate that an acid-base disorder is present.

If there are two or more acid-base disorders ("mixed acid-base disorder"), it is possible that the acidity of one buffers the alkalinity of the other, yielding, strangely, a pH in normal range.

Notes:

Section 93.0.1   <u>ACID-BASE DISORDER</u>
<u>DETERMINATIONS</u>

◊ Acid-base disorders are disorders that disrupt normal pH of the serum.
◊ Calculating acid-base requires the following steps:
    1. Determine if the pH is < 7.35 or > 7.45.
        If it is < 7.35, there is an acidemia (acidic blood).
        If it is > 7.45, there is an alkalemia (alkaline or basic blood)
    2. Look at HCO3 and pCO2. You are interested in comparing the measured value (from the patient) against the normal MEAN value for these components.
        Normal mean value of HCO3 = 24 mmol/mg
        Normal mean value of pCO2 = 40 mm Hg
    3. Determine if the HCO3 and pCO2 are trending higher than or lower than their normal mean values.
    4. If HCO3 and pCO2 are trending in the same direction as the pH, then it is a metabolic disorder.
    5. If pCO2 and pH are trending in opposite directions, then it is a respiratory disorder.
    6. Determine what type of respiratory or metabolic disorder it is by assigning its acid-base status (which was determined by the pH).

Example: Patient A has a blood pH of 7.30. HCO3 is 22 and pCO2 is 38. What acid-base disorder exists?

The pH is not within normal range (7.35-7.45), so we know that there is, indeed, an acid-base disorder present. The pH is lower than normal, so there is acidemia. That means we have to determine what type of acidosis this is. pH is trending down. HCO3 is trending down (from a normal mean of 24). pCO2 is trending down (from a normal mean of 40). So, both HCO3 and pCO2 are trending in the same direction as pH: down. Thus, this is a metabolic disorder, namely a metabolic acidosis.

- ◇ Now, you can calculate the expected compensation. To do that:
    1. First, you MUST figure out what type of acid-base disorder it is before trying to figure out compensation!! So, follow the previous instructions for doing that first.

        If it is a metabolic acidosis, use Winter's formula to determine the expected compensation:
        Expected $pCO_2 = (1.5 \times HCO_3) + 8 +/- 2$

        If it is metabolic alkalosis, use the following formula to determine the expected compensation:
        Expected $pCO_2 = (0.7 \times HCO_3) + 20 +/- 5$

        If it is respiratory acidosis that was of acute onset and short duration, the expected compensation will be that of HCO_3 being 1 mmol higher than normal mean for every 10 mm Hg increase in pCO_2 over normal mean.

        If it is respiratory acidosis that is of chronic and long duration, the expected compensation will be that of HCO_3 being 3-4 mmol higher than normal mean for every 10 mm Hg increase in pCO_2 over normal mean.

        If it is respiratory alkalosis that was of acute onset and short duration, the expected compensation will that of HCO_3 being 2 mmol lower than normal mean for every 10 mm Hg increase in pCO_2 over normal mean.

        If it is respiratory alkalosis that is of chronic and long duration, the expected compensation will be that of HCO_3 being 5 mm Hg lower than normal mean for every 10 mm Hg increase in pCO_2 over normal mean.

    2. Now, determine if the actual values of the patient fit within the expected compensation values.
    3. If the values are higher or lower than expected, that means that compensation has not occurred as expected BECAUSE there is a secondary acid-base disorder.

Boards Boot Camp High-Yield Compendium

For our previous patient with metabolic acidosis, let's see if there is expected compensation:

Patient A has a blood pH of 7.30. HCO3 is 22 and pCO2 is 39.
We have already determined that it is a metabolic acidosis. But, has compensation occurred as expected?

Expected pCO2 = (1.5 x HCO3) + 8 +/- 2 = (1.5 x 22) + 8 +/-2 = 41 +/- 2 = 39-43. Since the patient's pCO2 is 39, compensation has occurred as expected, meaning that there is no other additional acid-base disorder.

If, for example, his measured pCO2 had been, instead, 30, it would have been lower than expected. Since the patient has metabolic acidosis, but the pCO2 is lower than expected for normal compensation, the pCO2 could be getting blown off via respiration, such as with a respiratory alkalosis.

If, for example, his measured pCO2 had been, instead, 50, it would have been higher than expected, indicating that an additional acid-base disorder also exists, such as respiratory acidosis.

Section 93.0.2   <u>ACID-BASE DISORDERS</u>

Acid-Base Disorder	pH	HCO3	pCO2	Possible Causes
Metabolic acidosis	<7.35	⇓	⇓	Aspirin overdose Lactic acidosis DKA Diarrhea
		All trend downward		
Metabolic alkalosis	>7.45	⇑	⇑	Loop diuretics Thiazides Vomiting
		All trend upward		
Respiratory acidosis	<7.35	⇑	⇑	Sedation COPD Obstructive sleep apnea
		pCO2 trends in opposite direction of pH		
Respiratory alkalosis	>7.45	⇓	⇓	Panic attack Pain (causing hyperventilation)
		pCO2 trends in opposite direction of pH		

<u>Buffering Facts:</u>
Bicarbonate (HCO₃) is the most important buffer in the body.

Proteins, especially albumin, also have buffering actions by way of their weak acidic and basic groups within their structure. As such, intracellular proteins are particularly important in limiting pH changes <u>within cells</u>. Furthermore, the protein matrix of bones plays a critical role in buffering the plasma pH of patients with chronic acidosis.

Hemoglobin is, of course, important in ensuring delivery of oxygen to tissues. However, it also plays an important role in buffering. It does this through **its ability to bind both carbon dioxide (CO_2) and hydrogen ions (H^+),** an ability that is strongest when the hemoglobin is de-oxygenated. In fact, tissues take up oxygen delivered by hemoglobin, oxygen that allows them to undertake metabolism that yields the CO_2. That CO_2 is released by the cells, and either combines with water to produce carbonic acid or binds to the de-oxygenated hemoglobin (the Hb that brought the oxygen and that now is de-oxygenated). Upon return to the lung, the hemoglobin releases the CO2 into the alveoli, allowing its departure through the lung.

As for the CO_2 that becomes carbonic acid, the CO_2 released from the cells enters the RBCs and combines with water to, indeed, form carbonic acid. The reaction is catalyzed by carbonic anhydrase. But, then, the newly formed carbonic acid dissociates into bicarbonate and hydrogen ions. The hydrogen ions bind with hemoglobin while the bicarbonate leaves the RBC, entering the plasma. This bicarbonate is exchanged with chloride ions (Cl^-), allowing for chloride entry into the RBCs while the bicarbonate is exiting into the plasma. As for the hydrogen ions bound to the hemoglobin, they are brought to the lungs where they recombine with bicarbonate (which was released into the plasma by the RBC) to re-form carbon dioxide – and that carbon dioxide then exits via the lungs. At the same time, the hemoglobin binds oxygen, and the cycle begins.

Boards Boot Camp High-Yield Compendium

Thus, CO_2 **is effectively buffered by bicarbonate**, bicarbonate that is produced by and released from RBCs. Likewise, de-oxygenated hemoglobin also powerfully buffers carbon dioxide by binding it up, and delivering it to the lungs for removal.

Additionally, **hemoglobin can also bind hydrogen ions**, after which it delivers them to the lung for recombination with bicarbonate and formation of carbon dioxide that is removed by the lung.

The kidneys work to secrete hydrogen ions, thus allowing for elimination of hydrogen ions from the body. However, **kidneys also regenerate bicarbonate.**

Bicarbonate reaches the kidney via the blood, and is filtered by the glomerulus, allowing it to enter the renal tubules. However, most of it is reabsorbed back into the body in a process that occurs in the proximal convoluted tubule (PCT). What happens it the bicarbonate that reaches the PCT (after being filtered from the blood) combines with hydrogen ions in the PCT lumen. That combination yields carbonic acid, and is a reaction catalyzed by carbonic anhydrase. The carbonic acid in turn, in the lumen, dissociates to form carbon dioxide and water, both of which enter the renal tubule cells lining the PCT. Inside the renal tubular cells, the CO_2 recombines with the water, again under the actions of carbonic anhydrase, to form carbonic acid. And, that carbonic acid dissociates into bicarbonate and hydrogen ions. The bicarbonate enters the blood stream, and the hydrogen ions are released to the renal tubule lumen via a Na/H^+ exchange. Thus, the bicarbonate that is filtered out of the blood stream gets regenerated in the kidney, and returned to the blood stream. Additionally, as noted, hydrogen ions are secreted into the renal tubule for excretion.

Section 93.0.3   <u>Potassium and Acid-Base</u>

Cells provide tremendous buffering capacity in states of acidemia or alkalemia, but affect serum potassium levels as a result.

More than 50% of hydrogen ions in metabolic acidosis are actually buffered in cells.

In **metabolic acidosis**, cells function in a buffering capacity by transcellular exchange of hydrogen ions with potassium ions; the result is uptake of hydrogen ions into cells with movement of potassium to the extracellular environment. The result can be **hyperkalemia**.

The hyperkalemia that can result from metabolic acidosis accounts for the risk of arrhythmias with metabolic acidosis.

Conversely, in **metabolic alkalosis**, cells release hydrogen ions in exchange for uptake of potassium; the result is **hypokalemia**.

Similar, but much milder, effects can be seen with **respiratory acid-base disorders**.

Section 93.1   **FLUID SHIFTS**

ICV = intracellular volume; the volume of fluid in each RBC is the "standard" by which this is evaluated
ECV = extracellular volume; this is comprised of interstitial fluid and plasma. *⟵ not quantity*
Hct = hematocrit; the volume of blood occupied by RBC mass and is represented as a percentage of the total (e.g., normal hematocrit is generally around 45%)
Plasma = the fluid component of blood (and lymph)
Serum = plasma without fibrinogen (I)

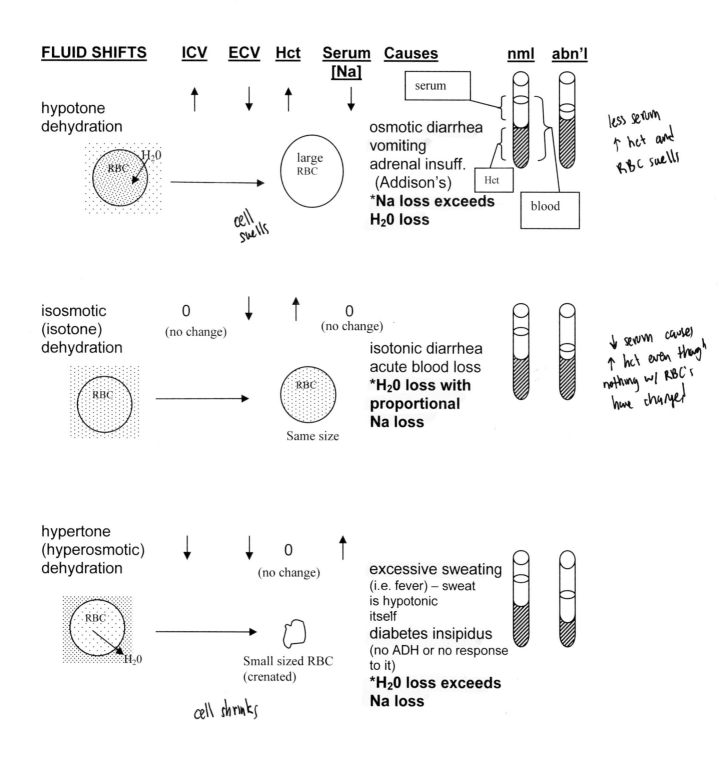

FLUID SHIFTS	ICV	ECV	Hct	Serum [Na]	Causes	nml	abn'l

hypotone dehydration — ICV ↑, ECV ↓, Hct ↑, Serum [Na] ↓

serum

osmotic diarrhea
vomiting
adrenal insuff.
(Addison's)
Na loss exceeds H_2O loss

Hct

blood

large RBC

cell swells

less serum ↑ hct and RBC swells

isosmotic (isotone) dehydration — ICV 0 (no change), ECV ↓, Hct ↑, Serum [Na] 0 (no change)

isotonic diarrhea
acute blood loss
H_2O loss with proportional Na loss

RBC — Same size

↓ serum causes ↑ hct even though nothing w/ RBC's have changed

hypertone (hyperosmotic) dehydration — ICV ↓, ECV ↓, Hct 0 (no change), Serum [Na] ↑

excessive sweating
(i.e. fever) – sweat is hypotonic itself
diabetes insipidus
(no ADH or no response to it)
H_2O loss exceeds Na loss

Small sized RBC (crenated)

cell shrinks

FLUID SHIFTS	ICV	ECV	Hct	Serum [Na]	Causes	nml	abn'l

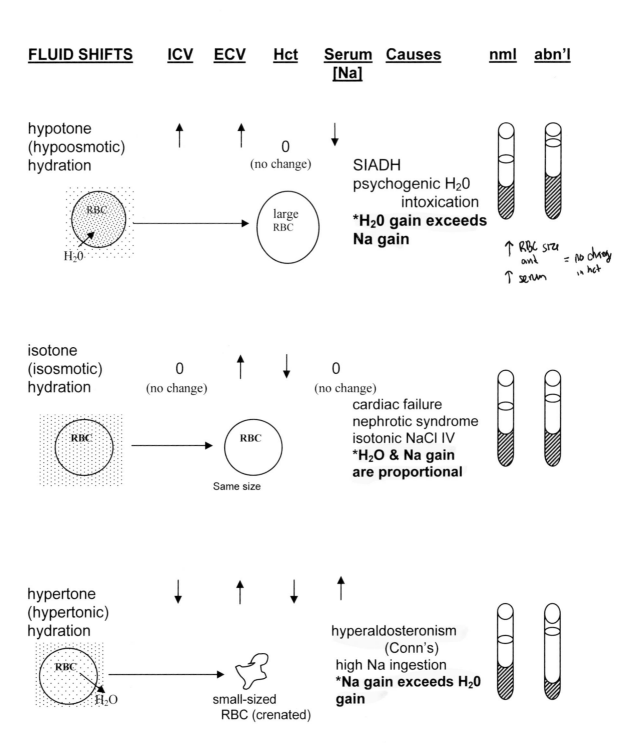

hypotone (hypoosmotic) hydration — ICV ↑, ECV ↑, Hct 0 (no change), Serum [Na] ↓

RBC + H₂O → large RBC

SIADH
psychogenic H₂0 intoxication
*H₂0 gain exceeds Na gain

↑ RBC size and ↑ serum = no change in hct

isotone (isosmotic) hydration — ICV 0 (no change), ECV ↑, Hct ↓, Serum [Na] 0 (no change)

RBC → RBC (Same size)

cardiac failure
nephrotic syndrome
isotonic NaCl IV
*H₂O & Na gain are proportional

hypertone (hypertonic) hydration — ICV ↓, ECV ↑, Hct ↓, Serum [Na] ↑

RBC → H₂O → small-sized RBC (crenated)

hyperaldosteronism (Conn's)
high Na ingestion
*Na gain exceeds H₂0 gain

Section 94.0   THE RAA SYSTEM
Renin-Angiotensin-Aldosterone System

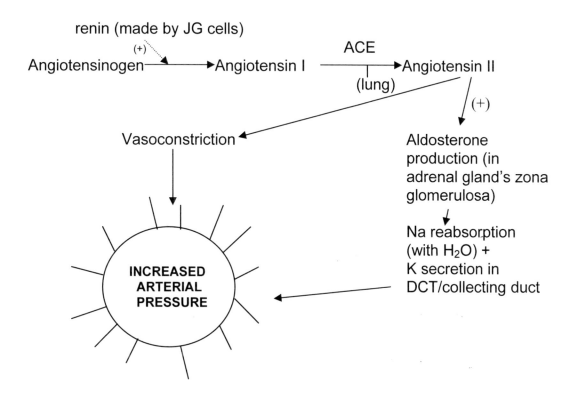

Section 95.0   UPPER GI TRACT
Includes the GI tract before the ligament of Treitz, and so contains the mouth, esophagus, stomach, the beginning portion of the duodenum

Section 95.1   MOUTH

Teeth are used to macerate the food, and saliva (secreted by the parotid, sublingual, and submandibular glands) contains alpha-amylase (which initiates starch digestion), mucins (which lubricate the food), and a pH that serves to neutralize bacterial acids (which decreases dental decay).

STOMACH

Chief Cells (in fundus and corpus)   produce pepsinogen

Parietal cells (in fundus, primarily)   produce HCl + intrinsic factor
(remember, PGs* decrease HCl secretion)

Mucus Cells (in fundus, corpus, & antrum)   produce mucus (remember, PGs*
increase mucus secretion)

G cells (in antrum)   produce gastrin   ↓ gastric emptying
stimulates Parietal cells

THE PARIETAL CELL

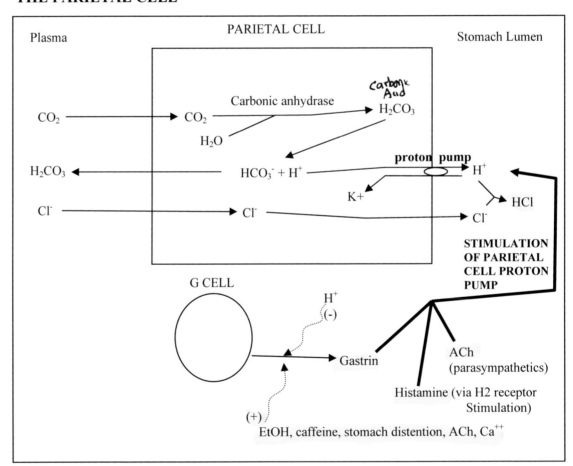

*PGs = prostaglandins

Section 96.0 GI HORMONES

	produced by:	*stimulants for release:*	*effects:*	
Gastrin	gastric G cells	PNS (ACh), peptides, EtOH, Ca, caffeine, stomach distention	parietal cell stimulation, decreased stomach emptying, increased stomach motility	
Secretin	S cells of duodenum	H ions in duodenum	HCO_3^- rich pancreatic Secretion	dont want acid in small intestine
CCK (cholecystokinin) to move	I cells of duodenum & jejunum	FAT (& fatty acids), peptides in duodenum & jejunum; PNS (ACh)	pancreatic EXOcrine activity (trypsinogen, etc.), gallbladder contractions	– melatonin seratonin niacin
GIP (gastric inhibitory protein)	duodenum & jejunum	glucose, fat, amino acid in duodenum & jejunum	stimulates insulin secretion by endocrine pancreas; inhibits gastric parietal cells	
Somatostatin	endocrine pancreas (delta cells)	H ions in duodenum (is inhibited by PNS)	inhibits gastric parietal cells; inhibits exocrine pancreas (enzymes); inhibits insulin & glucagon release by endocrine pancreas; inhibits growth hormone & thyroid hormone synthesis	
Vasoactive Intestinal Peptide (VIP)	smooth muscle cells & nervous tissue of intestine		relaxes intestinal smooth muscle, inhibits gastric acid secretion, & stimulates pancreatic bicarbonate secretion	

Section 96.1   <u>GI Absorption</u>

Molecule or Substance	Stomach	Duodenum	Jejunum	Ileum	Colon
Alcohol	X	X			
Carbohydrates		X	X		
Amino acids		X	X		
Bile salts				X	
Vitamin B12				X	
Water		X	X	X	X
Sodium			X	X	X
Bicarbonate			X	X	
Potassium			X	X	
Iron		X	X	X	X
Calcium		X	X	X	

- **Bile salts** are absorbed in the <u>terminal</u> ileum.

- **Vitamin B12** absorption occurs in the <u>terminal</u> ileum.

- Approximately 90% of the **water** in feces/chyme is absorbed by the small intestine; the remaining 10% is absorbed by the colon.

- **Sodium** absorption in the jejunum is absorbed mostly via co-transport, as a result of active uptake of sugars and amino acids (it is a process like that seen for Na uptake at the proximal convoluted tubule).

- Sodium is actively absorbed in the ileum and the colon.

Boards Boot Camp High-Yield Compendium

- **Bicarbonate** absorption occurs in the jejunum via a process mediated by active secretion of hydrogen ions (this mechanism resembles the mechanism for bicarbonate absorption in the proximal convoluted tubule).

- Ileal absorption of HCO3 (bicarbonate) only occurs if luminal concentrations of bicarbonate are excessive.

- Interestingly, if bicarbonate luminal concentrations (e.g., in the intestine) are very low, the ileum and colon will *secrete* more bicarbonate into the intestine!

- **Potassium** undergoes passive absorption in the jejunum and ileum.

- Interestingly, the colon typically secretes potassium mostly passively. This explains why tremendous potassium loss tends to occur with diarrhea (e.g., since the secretion is passive, it depends on electrochemical gradients; in diarrhea, ions are diluted by the water content of the stool, making for a greater gradient from extraluminal to intraluminal environs, encouraging the movement of potassium into the colonic lumen and eventual loss with stool).

- Even without diarrhea, stool represents a major vehicle by which potassium is removed from the body (the other vehicle is urine).

- **Iron** is mostly absorbed in the duodenum and proximal jejunum, although any part of the intestine is capable of absorbing small amounts of reduced iron.

- In the intestine, **non-heme iron** (iron not acquired from meat) binds to receptors on the brush border of the enterocytes (cells lining the bowel); the receptor numbers increase at times of iron deficiency. **Heme iron** (iron acquired from meat) is absorbed directly without receptors, and released to the blood stream. Non-heme iron, instead, associates with ferritin intracellularly. From there, iron is transferred to outside of the cell, wherein it binds transferrin for transport through the blood and in all interstitial spaces. Transferrin exchanges iron with all cells of the body. Any iron still bound to ferritin in the enterocyte is lost when that cell sloughs off.

- Iron absorption is increased in the presence of **vitamin C, alcohol, and fructose**

- Iron absorption is decreased in the presence of **dietary fiber, calcium and calcium-containing foods (e.g., milk), as well as tea or coffee.**

- **Calcium** is absorbed in the duodenum and proximal jejunum via an active vitamin D-dependent process, and is absorbed in the ileum via mostly a passive vitamin D-independent process.

- An increase in calcium absorption is stimulated by **parathyroid hormone (PTH), growth hormone, and insulin.**

- Calcium absorption is inhibited by **cortisol, thyroxine (thyroid hormone), and glucagon.**

Boards Boot Camp High-Yield Compendium

- The main absorptive and secretory role of the **colon** is that of absorbing water, Na, Cl and secreting K and HCO3. Most of the water it absorbs is absorbed in the ascending and transverse colon, accounting for the semi-solid character of feces in the descending colon. Water absorption in the colon is decreased by ADH (like the effects seen in the collecting duct of the kidney) and by inflammation.

Section 97.0   ADRENAL HORMONES

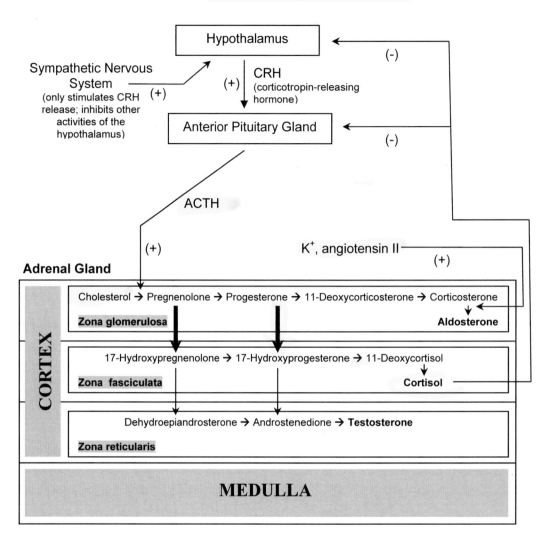

When the adrenal gland is stimulated by **ACTH**, cholesterol is converted to pregnenolone, but then the conversion of pregnenolone to 17-hydroxypregnenolone and the conversion of progesterone to 17-hydroxyprogesterone is HIGHLY favored over the terminal reactions of the zona glomerulosa. The result is that ACTH release causes a pronounced **cortisol** production and release. So, while ACTH is necessary for aldosterone production, it is the least important factor in determining the amounts of **aldosterone** that are made. In fact, the two most important factors in determining aldosterone manufacture are **potassium ions** and **angiotensin II**, both of which act as strong stimulators to aldosterone synthesis.

An extremely potent stimulator to hypothalamic release of **CRH** is the **sympathetic nervous system**. This is unusual, since other aspects of hypothalamic activity generally are inhibited under the influence of the sympathetic nervous system. In fact, it is the sympathetic nervous system's

569

inhibitory influence over the hypothalamus that is responsible for amenorrhea in females who are very emotionally **stressed**, **critically ill**, or suffering from **anorexia nervosa**.

Under stress, emotional and physical, the hypothalamus is therefore stimulated to produce and release CRH which, in turn, stimulates the anterior pituitary gland to manufacture and release ACTH. The ACTH then acts on the adrenal gland, launching an increase in adrenocortical hormone synthesis with STRONG preference for cortisol. This is why cortisol is termed the "**stress hormone**," as it is produced rapidly and in large quantities while one is under stress. In turn, cortisol has many effects.

Cortisol Effects   *Stress*

1. Stimulation of gluconeogenesis
2. Increase in insulin resistance
3. Increase in glycogenesis
4. Increase in serum glucose levels (hyperglycemia)
5. Mobilization of amino acids from mostly skeletal muscle
6. Decrease in protein synthesis (except as noted below)
7. Increase in production of proteins, including enzymes, in the liver
8. Mobilization of fatty acids from adipose tissue (increase in lipolysis)
9. Increase in serum lipid levels (hyperlipidemia)
10. Increase in food intake (mechanism not fully understood)
11. Inhibition of prostaglandin production (thus, decreases fever and other inflammatory effects)
12. Stabilization of cellular lysosomes, so that damaged cells do not as readily release tissue-destructive enzymes that usually reside in these lysosomes
13. Decrease in capillary permeability (causing decreased edema and swelling)
14. Decrease in chemotaxis
15. Decrease in T cell production (resulting in lymphocytopenia)
16. Decrease in antibody production
17. Increase in RBC production (and possible polycythemia
18. Increase in neutrophil production (and neutrocytosis)
19. Decrease in IL-1 production and release (thus decreases macrophage generated immune responses and decreases fever)
20. Upregulate alpha 1 receptors, increasing vasoconstrictive effect of norepinephrine and resulting in increased blood pressure.
21. Decrease in osteoblast activity

This preference for the production of cortisol, rather than other adrenocortical hormones, when stimulated by ACTH accounts for the features of Cushing's disease, wherein the pituitary gland produces excess quantities of ACTH with a resulting excess production of primarily cortisol.

Section 97.1   Addison's Disease

Addison's disease = hypoaldosteronism = primary adrenal insufficiency

Because there is no aldosterone acting on the kidney:
1.   Hyponatremia (due to Na loss)
2.   Hypotension (due to Na loss)
3.   Hyperkalemia (because there is no Na/K exchange)
4.   H ion retention (therefore, metabolic acidosis) (because there's no K/H exchange)
5.   Hypoglycemia (because there will also often be lower than normal levels of cortisol)
6.   Pigmentation...why? Decreased aldosterone production in this disease is also associated with decreased cortisol production, resulting in no negative feedback on the anterior pituitary. So, there is VERY high ACTH that is produced (but ACTH is part of a larger precursor molecule that is made by the anterior pituitary):

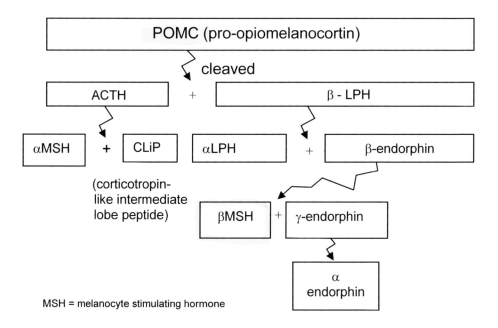

MSH = melanocyte stimulating hormone

The excess ACTH that is produced comes from an excess in POMC production. Excess POMC production results in excess MSH production, causing hyperpigmentation of the skin due to stimulation by the MSH of melanocytes.

Section 98.0   HORMONES OF THE ANTERIOR PITUITARY GLAND

Corticotropin, also known as ACTH (adrenocorticotropic hormone), works to stimulate the adrenal cortex. It has no influence over the adrenal medulla, the site of production of norepinephrine and epinephrine destined to be released directly to the blood stream.

Gonadotrope hormones are hormones that stimulate the gonads (ovaries and testes). They include FSH (follicle stimulating hormone) and LH (luteinizing hormone).

Thyrotropin hormone works to stimulate the thyroid gland. It is manufactured by thyrotropes and is termed "Thyroid Stimulating Hormone" or TSH.

Growth hormone is produced by somatotropes, and stimulates body growth and increased serum glucose levels.

Prolactin is produced by lactotropes and works to stimulate breast tissue for milk production.

#1 = prolactinoma

NOTE: The posterior pituitary gland does not produce hormones, but instead secretes hormones made by the hypothalamus; those include ADH (anti-diuretic hormone; vasopressin) which works to stimulate water reabsorption from the kidney, and oxytocin which stimulates uterine contraction and milk release from the breast.

Insufficient secretion of ADH results in diabetes insipidus, a disorder which features polyuria and polydipsia. Excessive secretion of ADH causes SIADH, syndrome of inappropriate ADH, a disorder that features hyponatremia (due to water retention, so Na is diluted) with concomitant mental status changes (due to hyponatremia). Either disorder can occur as a result to head trauma, among other causes such as meningitis. *(FYI: There are two types of diabetes insipidus: central, which is due to insufficient secretion, and nephrogenic, which is inherited and due to lack of response by kidney to ADH).*

in collecting duct

Section 98.1

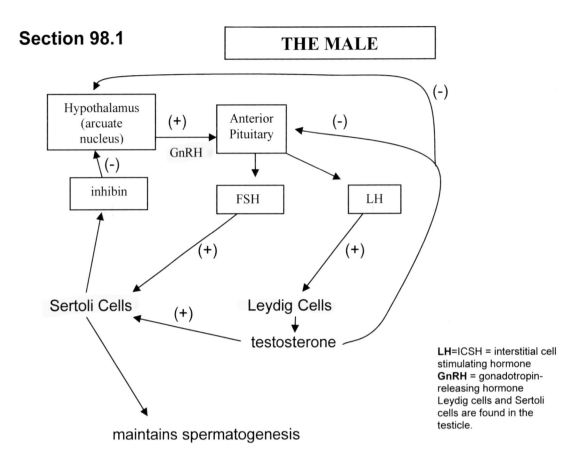

LH=ICSH = interstitial cell
stimulating hormone
GnRH = gonadotropin-
releasing hormone
Leydig cells and Sertoli
cells are found in the
testicle.

Section 98.1.0   ERECTION and ERECTILE DYSFUNCTION

→ Erection integrates processes involving the CNS, the peripheral nervous system, hormones, and the vascular system.

→ Tumescence = vascular filling of the penile cavernous bodies, creating erection

→ The extent of corpus cavernosal smooth muscle contraction is what determines the erectile state of the penis.

→ Factors that mediate smooth muscle contraction in the penis, promoting flaccidity, are norepinephrine, endothelin-1, and angiotensin II.

→ Factors that mediate relaxation of smooth muscle in the *Part: Pan* penis, promoting erection, include acetylcholine (ACh), nitric oxide (NO), and ATP.

→ As the corpora cavernosa tissue fills and expands, the venules under the rigid tunica albuginea become compressed. This results in nearly complete obstruction to venous outflow from the penis.

→ The bulbocavernosus reflex occurs with further sexual stimulation, forcing the ischiocavernosus muscles to compress the base of the blood-filled corpora cavernosa. It is at this point that the penis reaches full erection, since both inflow and outflow of blood is temporarily ceased.

   o The bulbocavernosus reflex has been shown to be delayed or absent in a higher proportion of diabetic men and circumcised men with complaints of impotence.

→ Nitric oxide (NO) is of particularly critical important to gaining and maintaining an erection. Most drugs currently used for ED operate on this principle.

→ NO is produced by nitric oxide synthase (NOS) via the oxidation of arginine. In the corpora cavernosum, NO activates guanylate cyclase, yielding increased levels of cGMP. cGMP causes vascular smooth muscle relaxation, allowing for, in the penis, blood filling and erection.

→ Phosphodiesterase then metabolizes cGMP.

→ ED meds are inhibitors of phosphodiesterase-5 (PDE-5), the enzyme that metabolizes cGMP associated with erection. No cGMP metabolism means higher cGMP levels, and increased erection potential along with prolonged erection potential.

→ These PDE-5 inhibitors include sildenafil, vardenafil, and others.

→ Interestingly, studies have also shown improvement with ED after just oral administration of arginine (the substrate for NO production).

→ NO has also been demonstrated to affect sexual behavior, and not just erection, by acting at the medial preoptic area and the paraventricular nucleus. Thus, it is thought to also potentiate successful sexual activity by also promoting desire plus hormonal inducement (via oxytocin production) of erection.

→ ED can by psychogenic or organic.

→ There are many diseases that can promote ED because of their effect on vasculature, hormones, and nervous system.

→ Diseases and drugs that place men at higher risk for ED are:

Atherosclerosis (MI, PVD)
Hypertension
Diabetes mellitus
Scleroderma
Liver cirrhosis
CVA
MS
Alzheimer's disease
COPD
Hyperthyroidism
Hypothyroidism
Pheochromocytoma
Depression
PTSD
Sickle cell anemia
Brain and spinal cord injury

Radical prostatectomy
Transurethral resection of the prostate
    (TURP)
Antihypertensives
Antidepressants
Antipsychotics
5-alpha reductase inhibitors

→ Detumescence occurs following cGMP metabolization, a
   process that occurs following sympathetic nervous system
   activation that is associated with ejaculation.

THE FEMALE

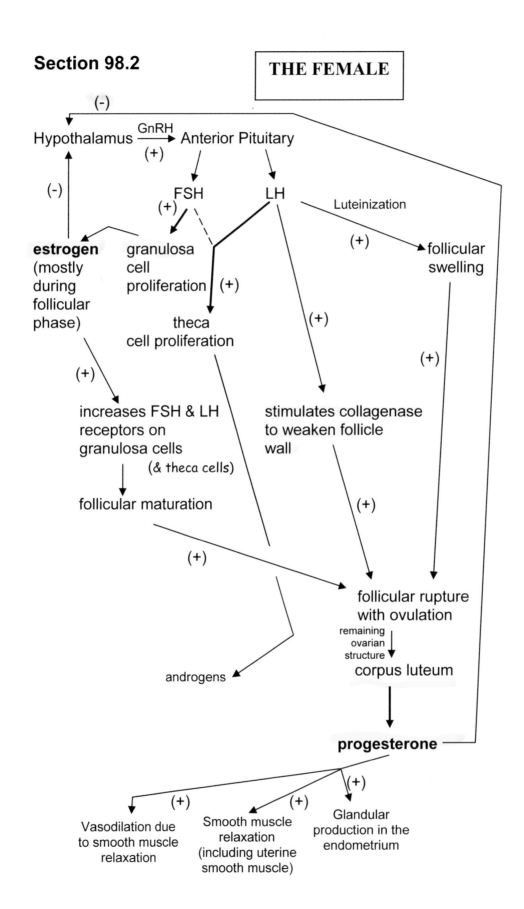

Boards Boot Camp High-Yield Compendium

Section 98.2.1   Female Menstrual Cycle Hormones

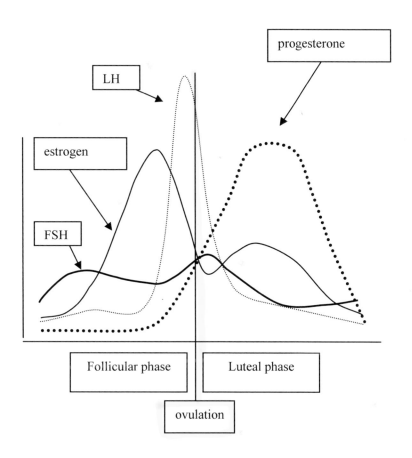

Section 98.3   DETAILS OF
FEMALE REPRODUCTIVE SYSTEM

The hypothalamus releases gonadotropin-releasing hormone (GnRH) →
stimulates anterior pituitary to secrete luteinizing hormone (LH) and follicle
stimulating hormone (FSH).
    1) The hypothalamic secretions must be pulsatile to have this effect.
    2) GnRH release is inhibited by estrogen and progesterone.

LH → development and maintenance of corpus luteum in ovary

FSH → development of follicle in ovary

Estrogens and progesterones are secreted by the follicles (estrogen only) and
the corpus luteum (both hormones, but MOSTLY progesterone).

578

Section 98.3.1   THE FEMALE MENSTRUAL CYCLE

The Cycle:

1) Estrogen and progesterone levels are low

2) Because estrogen and progesterone levels are low, there is no negative inhibition on the hypothalamus, so the hypothalamus releases GnRH.

3) GnRH stimulates the anterior pituitary to release FSH and LH.

4) FSH stimulates 12-14 primary ovarian follicles to undergo maturation

A)   Each follicle is surrounded by granulosa cells; these cells begin to secret fluid and estrogen into the center of the follicle
B)   The fluid-filled follicular center expands to become an antrum that surrounds the contained oocyte = this whole structure is known as an antral follicle
C)   The estrogen in the antrum begins to diffuse into the bloodstream, thereby increasing serum levels of estrogen
D)   The process continues because of continued stimulation by FSH
E)   The granulosa cells continue to proliferate while a surrounding layer of theca cells develop
F)   Eventually the developing follicle is referred to as a vesicular follicle.
G)   After a total of one week of follicular development, one follicle starts to outgrow the others – the other follicles undergo atresia and degenerate.
H)   The remaining follicle continues to grow and develop rapidly, with continued proliferation of theca and granulosa cells; this is stimulated by FSH as well as, indirectly, estrogen
→ estrogen stimulates the development of more LH and FSH receptors on the granulosa and theca cells, making them more responsive to those hormones

5) Eventually a high concentration of estrogen is attained in the blood stream which, then, serves to inhibit GnRH release from the hypothalamus.

6) LH and FSH release from the anterior pituitary then slows

7) At about day 12 of the cycle, the anterior pituitary produces a surge of LH (exact mechanism is unknown).

8) The LH surge then heralds the beginning of progesterone production by the theca cells and a proteolytic enzyme into the antrum.

9) At an area of the follicular wall, a weakness develops due to the proteolytic enzyme. This develops near the surface of the ovary. Eventually the follicle ruptures, releasing its contents: an oocyte covered in layers of granulosa cells.
→ this process occurs within 16 hours after the LH surge

10) The remaining ruptured follicle tissue in the ovary still contains layers of granulosa cells and theca cells. These cells were converted to lutein cells by the LH surge that occurred just before ovulation. In this process, they become engorged and yellowed.

11) The structure created by the lutein cells is known as the corpus luteum.

12) The granulosa cells of the corpus luteum produce large quantities of progesterone and smaller quantities of estrogen. The theca cells of the corpus luteum produce androstenedione and testosterone. Most of these androgenic hormones are converted to estrogens by granulosa cells.

13) After the LH surge, LH levels gradually decrease.

14) As long as LH remains in the bloodstream, it still has an activating effect on the granulosa and theca cells of the corpus luteum; hence, they continue to produce estrogens, progesterones, and testosterones.

15) After 12 days (very consistently 12 days from woman to woman), the LH level is so low that it no longer has any stimulating effect on the corpus luteum; the greatest determinant of this is the negative feedback that the estrogen and progesterone have on the hypothalamus such that estrogen and progesterone levels become so high that no GnRH is released, and, consequently, no LH is produced.

16) The corpus luteum degenerates and stops making hormones.

17) Within 2 days after the corpus luteum begins degeneration, menstruation begins.

18) At the same time as menstruation begins, FSH and LH begin to rise secondary to increasing GnRH levels (which, themselves, rise secondary to low estrogen and progesterone levels).

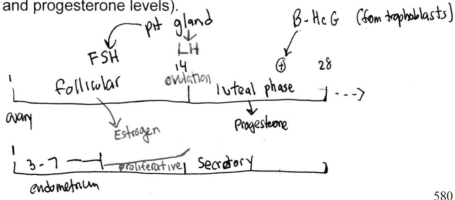

Boards Boot Camp High-Yield Compendium

Section 98.3.2   Estrogen

- stimulates the growth and development of the uterus, external female sex organs, and the breasts; it also stimulates osteoblasts to build bone.
- causes proliferation of endometrial cells (the epithelial cells that line the inner cavity of the uterus).

Section 98.3.3   Progesterone

- promotes "secretory" changes in the endometrium during the latter half of the menstrual cycle; it has a similar effect on the fallopian tube cells.
- the secretory function means that it encourages the development of glandular structures that support the structure of the endometrium and that secrete a fluid that provides nutrition for the fertilized ovum.
- reduces the motility and contractility of uterine smooth muscle (which is helpful since, during pregnancy, progesterone levels are exceptionally high)
- progesterone also inhibits smooth muscle elsewhere; during pregnancy, it is responsible for constipation and reflux
- stimulates the development of the lobules of the breast
- increases basal body temperature

Section 98.3.4   The Monthly Cycle of the Endometrium

1)   Elevated estrogen (produced from developing follicles – specifically from their granulosa cells) serves to cause endometrial cell proliferation.

2)   Within 4-7 days of menstruation, the entire endometrial surface is re-epithelialized.

3)   During the remaining days prior to menstruation, the continued estrogenic stimulation causes increased thickening of the endometrial layer (causing it to get as much as 4 mm thick at this point!)

4)   Steps 1-3 are the "proliferate phase", because it is the phase in which the endometrial cells proliferate; the remaining steps constitute the "secretory phase," a phase marked by secretory gland development.

5)   After ovulation, the corpus luteum secretes some estrogen in addition to tremendously high levels of progesterone.

6)   The progesterone stimulates glandular development in the endometrial layer, and causes the endometrial cells to accumulate lipids and glycogen in their cytoplasm. The stimulated glands secrete nutritive fluid for the zygote.

7)   The vascularity of the endometrium continues to grow to meet the growing demands of the new tissue.

581

8)   About 1 week after ovulation, the endometrium with its endometrial cells and glandular structures grow to a thickness of about 6 mm.

9)   At 12 days after ovulation, the corpus luteum degenerates and fails to manufacture any further estrogen and progesterone.

10)   Within 2 days of that, the endometrial involutes; within 24 hours of that process, the blood vessels serving the endometrium become vasospastic and the endometrium itself becomes ischemic and necrotic.

11)   The endometrial layer is shed, resulting in menses. Elevated levels of prostaglandin E allow for some uterine contractions to aid in ridding of the necrotic tissue. Low levels of progesterone also contribute to the stimulation of uterine contractions.

Section 98.3.5   FSH versus LH Levels

PUBERTY   hi FSH, hi LH   little Estrogen

MENOPAUSE   hi FSH, hi LH, but FSH levels are two times or more higher than those of LH

PCOS   lo FSH, hi LH with LH levels 2 times or more higher than FSH

Section 98.3.6   ANOVULATION
the lack of ovulation

Reasons for failure to ovulate:
→mechanical obstruction of the ovary
        - thickened capsule
        - scarring from infection
        - endometriosis, with endometrial cells blocking the ovulation process
→ absence of LH surge (e.g. menopause)

Sometimes, the inability to conceive is not due to anovulation. Fallopian tube pathology can be a cause, as well.

Reasons for obstructed fallopian tubes, leading to infertility:
→ scarring from infection (PID)
→ endometriosis, with obstructing endometrial cells

Section 98.3.7   <u>PREGNANCY</u>

Fertilization takes place in the fallopian tube (oviduct).

> → before fertilization can take place, the corona radiata (the outer layers of granulosa cells) must be removed by the actions of many sperm which release proteolytic enzymes (which are released from the acrosome of the sperm).
> → then, one sperm binds to and penetrates the zona pellucida

A fertilized ovum is a zygote.

The zygote takes 3-4 days to travel through the fallopian tube. While in the fallopian tube, the zygote becomes a blastocyst. Then, the blastocyst remains unattached in the uterus for another 3 days. At about 7 days total after fertilization, the trophoblast cells on the outer surface of the blastocyst start to release proteolytic enzymes. These enzymes digest and liquefy underlying endometrium, allowing the blastocyst to invade and attach to the endometrium.

The trophoblast cells produce human chorionic gonadotropin (beta-hCG). hCG enters the bloodstream and binds to LH receptors on the cells of the corpus luteum. Therefore, even though LH levels are decreasing, the hCG serves, by way of LH receptor binding, to cause stimulation of the LH receptors. Hence, the corpus luteum is maintained and, as such, continues to elaborate some estrogen as well as very large amounts of progesterone. The estrogen and, especially, the progesterone then serve to maintain the endometrial lining in a viable state for the developing embryo. Likewise, because of the hCG effect on the corpus luteum (and the resulting maintenance of the endometrium), menstruation does not occur.

Also, hCG binds to LH receptors on the Leydig cells in the testes of male fetuses. This stimulates the Leydig cells to produce testosterone, a process necessary for normal male differentiation during embryonic development.

Eventually, the placenta with its trophoblast cells manufactures the necessary estrogen and progesterone – and does so at very large levels, especially with regard to the progesterone!

The estrogen serves to, besides its effect on maintaining endometrium:
Enlarge mother's uterus
Enlarge mother's breasts, along with development of ducts
Enlarge mother's external genitalia

The progesterone, besides its effect on maintaining endometrium, serves to:
Encourage breast alveolar development
Reduce uterine contractility
Encourage storage of nutrients in the endometrial cells, converting them into nutritive decidual cells

583

Parturition is the process of birth of the baby. In the 7th month of pregnancy, progesterone levels continue to be high, but estrogen levels grow even higher. Estrogen has stimulatory effects on the contractility of the uterus. In the final weeks just prior to delivery, the levels of estrogen surge, creating a very contractile uterus.

Also, during the final weeks of pregnancy, the number of oxytocin receptors on the uterine smooth muscle cells increase. Oxytocin is secreted by the posterior pituitary gland. During labor, the levels of oxytocin rise sharply, causing strong uterine contractions.

Additionally, stretch of the uterus and cervix also makes it more contractile.

Spontaneous abortion = loss of fetus before the 20th week of gestation
There are 5 types of spontaneous abortion: threatened, inevitable, completed, incomplete, and missed. All result in fetal demise except for threatened, which only involves bleeding but no loss or passage of fetus or fetal parts.

Preterm delivery = birth of infant between 20 weeks and 36 weeks of gestation

Term delivery = birth of infant at 37-41weeks gestation

Post-term delivery = birth of infant beyond 42 weeks gestation

Infant maturity occurs at about 32-33 weeks gestation. Prematurity is associated with risk for infant acute respiratory distress syndrome, necrotizing enterocolitis, and a range of other disorders associated with lack of maturity of organs and organ systems for normal function.

Infants born before 32-33 weeks gestational age are considered premature. All premature infants are preterm, but not all preterm infants are premature.

Section 98.4　　　　　　**THYROID FUNCTION**

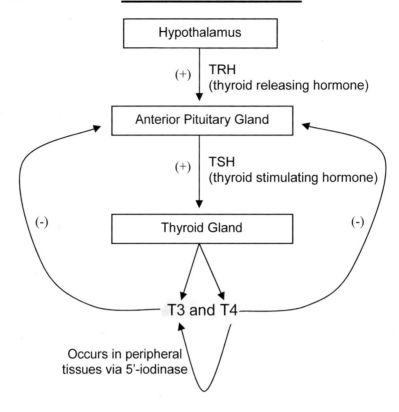

- T3 is four times more biologically active than T4.

- Regardless of TSH stimulation, high levels of I⁻ inhibit thyroid hormone synthesis, resulting in decreased thyroid hormone production and hypothyroidism; this is known as the Wolff-Chaikoff effect.

- The effects of the thyroid hormones (T3 and T4) include growth (particularly bony development and maturation), CNS maturation (during the perinatal period), anxiety and irritability, up-regulation of beta-one receptors on the heart (causing increased heart rate, stroke volume, and cardiac output), decreased protein metabolism, increased glycogenolysis, gluconeogenesis, and glycolysis, increased lipolysis (e.g., weight loss), increased glucose absorption from the bowel, increased respiration rate, and increased oxygen consumption because of increased metabolism in all tissues except the testicles, ovaries, brain, and spleen (which accounts for the hyperthermia at times of hyperthyroidism).

Todd's paralysis
- stroke like
symptom after
seizure

Epilepsy: A <u>recurrent paroxysmal</u> disorder of cerebral function characterized by severe, brief attacks of altered consciousness, motor activity, sensory phenomena, and abnormal behavior caused by abnormal excessive discharge of cerebral neurons → seizures. There is <u>no identifiable acute cause</u>.

Note: Not all people who have seizures are epileptic ("primary epilepsy"). Seizures also occur in persons with brain pathology, such as brain tumors, increased intracerebral pressures, meningitis/encephalitis, CVAs, aneurysms, hemorrhages into or around brain (subarachnoid, epidural, subdural, intracranial), etc. Thus, seizure disorder can be a manifestation of a serious CNS disorder.

Complex seizure causes loss of consciousness
Simple seizure does not cause loss of consciousness
Partial seizure affects only one part of the brain
Generalized seizure affects the entire brain
Seizure is the electrical overactivity in the brain
Convulsion is the motor effect that some seizures have on the body

Grand Mal = a type of generalized complex seizure
　　　　　　　Tonic/clonic movement (convulsion), loss of consciousness, incontinence;
　　　　　　　May have auras (sensory perceptions) just prior to the event
　　　　　　　Will have post-ictal state (confused, lethargic) after seizure
　　　　　　　High voltage spikes on EEG

Petit Mal = Absence Seizure
　　　　　　　A generalized complex seizure
　　　　　　　A special type of seizure characterized by 10-30 seconds of loss of consciousness where the patient remains immobile with eyes either staring or eyelids fluttering; patient usually remains seated or standing during the event as there is no loss of muscle tone
　　　　　　　3/sec spike and dome on EEG
　　　　　　　Occurs only in children
　　　　　　　Usually self-resolves, and is not associated with brain pathology
　　　　　　　Treated with ethosuxomide (alternate is valproic acid)

Febrile Seizures　　Never associated with epilepsy
　　　　　　　Occurs secondary to fever in children < 6 years old
　　　　　　　Treatment is not geared towards "seizure treatment;" management is focused on reducing fever and finding and eliminating the cause of the fever

Psychomotor Seizure = a complex generalized, complex partial, or simple partial seizure

A "temporal lobe seizure"

If simple, partial: Patient does not lose consciousness – but there is a change in behavior, and patient complains of feeling strange, of hallucinating unpleasant odors or tastes, of having feelings of déjà vu, and of frequently encountering "religious" experiences

If complex generalized, patient will lose consciousness; complex partial seizures of this type often occur in concert with automatisms and sitting or walking about aimlessly – and this is usually accompanied by hand wringing, lip smacking, profuse sweating, flushing, and borborygmi. The patient performs automatic purposeless movements or utters unintelligible sounds

→ lip smacking, staggering, shaking head

Lasts 1-2 minutes with confusion (if not generalized), then quickly resolves

Spikes in temporal lobe on EEG

Myoclonic seizure = a simple generalized seizure

Features jerks, head nods – all usually minor and only few in number for each episode

There is no loss of consciousness

Jacksonian Seizure = a type of simple focal seizure

Movements start in one focal area, and then spread to neighboring areas (this corresponds to the spread of seizure activity in the brain)

Increased electrical activity around antral sulcus on EEG

Section 100.0   SOCIAL SCIENCE

Section 100.1   Conditioning

Conditioning   Classical = Pavlovian =   involuntary (lost if not continually conditioned)

Operant = Cognitive Conditioning = voluntary response (the conditioned response has "resistance to extinction" → the person is less likely to change if conditioned in this way)

Section 100.2   Developmental Milestones

Birth: Cries, kicks legs
6 weeks: Raises chin when prone, smiles at others
2 months: Holds head steady when held sitting, reaches out
             when prone, tugs at clothing, makes cooing sounds
4 months: Rolls from front to back, pulls objects to mouth,
             laughs
5 months: Moro reflex disappears
6 months: Ulnar grasping, responds to name, starts babbling,
             stranger anxiety
7 months: Sits without support, stands with help
8 months: Crawls on stomach, says ma-ma, da-da
             indiscriminately
9 months: Can pull oneself up to stand, separation anxiety
10 months: Can stand alone holding on to furniture
11 months: Stands alone without support, uses ma-ma and da-da
             specifically for parents
1 year: Walks with support, pincer grasp, throws things,
             Babinski starts to disappear, drinks with sippy cup,
             says one word clearly (besides ma-ma and da-da)
14 months: Stands alone
15 months: Walks without support, draws lines, points to
             wanted items, speaks sounds in tandem "like"
             sentences
18 months: Climbs steps with support, can scribble, uses spoon,
             uses 5-10 words and is able to say own name
2 years: Runs, kicks ball, Babinski has disappeared, undresses
             self, speaks 2-word sentences, exhibits parallel play,
             might be ready to start toilet training (beware: not all
             children are ready by this age, and should not be forced to
             do so until ready)

3 years: Rides tricycle, can copy a circle, dresses and undresses self successfully (except for buttons), able to use toilet or potty chair but needs help with wiping

4 years: Can hop on 1 foot, can copy a cross, able to tell a story, exhibits cooperative play, fully toilet trained, able to button clothes

5 years: Skips, catches ball, can copy a square, able to print own name, ties shoelaces, speaks fluently (although some things may be mispronounced)

6 years: Rides bicycle, can copy a triangle, begins to read, may start to use knife

- Differences can be seen in reported **"standards" in developmental milestones** as some represent the mean value, the median value, the youngest age, or the oldest age (beyond which there is concern of developmental delay). So realize that, although a firm age is reported in any developmental milestone chart or list, these are values that actually sit within a range of what is considered normal.

- The **moro reflex** is a normal reflex in infants ages newborn to about 4-5 months of age. It is a response to a sudden loss of support that makes the infant feel like he is falling. The reflex includes, in order, arm abduction, then arm adduction, and, usually, crying. Absence of the reflex indicates profound motor system pathology. A unilateral absence or defect in the reflex indicates brachial plexus injury, hemiplegia, or a fracture clavicle. Likewise, persistence beyond 5 months of age is noted in infants with several neurologic problems, such as cerebral palsy.

- The **Babinski sign** is normal in newborns, and disappears sometime between their 1st and 2nd birthday. It is a result of the as-yet incompletely myelinated corticospinal tract of the spinal cord, a normal finding in infants up to 2 years of age.

IQ tests assess intelligence. The standard IQ test median is 100. Anyone with an IQ less than 70 is deemed to have intellectual disability. An IQ of 55-70 represents mild intellectual disability (educable), 40-55 indicates moderate intellectual disability (able to be trained to maintain personal hygiene), 25-40 is representative of severe intellectual disability, and those with an IQ less than 25 are considered profoundly intellectually disabled. Those with severe MR/ID or profound MR/ID generally require custodial care 24/7.

Section 100.3   <u>**The 5 Stages of Grief**</u>
as described by Elisabeth Kubler-Ross

Denial
Anger
Bargaining
Depression
Acceptance

Dr. Kubler-Ross notes that these stages occur in <u>NO</u> particular order (e.g., can occur in any order), and not everyone will experience all stages. She holds that these 5 stages of grief are common reactions to serious illness, death, and loss of any type (news of a terminal illness, children in divorce, love-interest break up, loss of job or home, loss of bodily function (disability), etc)

Section 100.3   <u>**Substance Use Disorders**</u>

➢ **Abuse** = use that results in problems at work, school, or home, OR legal problems, OR that creates dangerous situations.

➢ **Dependence** = recurrent and persistent use of drugs because the drug is needed for normal function; abruptly stopping leads to withdrawal

➢ **Tolerance** = the need to continually increase dosage to obtain same desired effect of drug; is because of the body's physical adaptation to the effects of the drug.

➢ **Addiction** = psychological attachment to a drug, featuring chronic, recurring compulsive drug seeking and use, despite harmful consequences. Addiction is, therefore, characterized by an intense impulse to take drugs.

Imaging studies in addicts typically demonstrate changes in brain architecture, particularly changes in areas critical to judgment, decision making, learning, memory, and behavioral control.

- A patient can have a physical dependence without having an addiction. Examples:

  Opioid analgesics. A patient using these for pain relief may become physically dependent, but is unlikely to become addicted if treatment is managed appropriately

- A patient can have an addiction without having physical dependence, since addiction is the psychological compulsion to use that drug, whereas dependence is the physiologic need to use it to maintain normal function.
- Drug abuse can lead to dependence and/or addiction.

Common Drugs of Abuse

Substance	Street names	Intoxication	Withdrawal
Cocaine	Coke, blow, bump, candy, Charlie, rock, snow	Increased confidence & energy, euphoria, dilated pupils, with risk of MI, CVA, cardiac arrest, seizure	Apathy, intense depression, fatigue
Alcohol	Booze, hooch, red-eye, hair of the dog, brew (for beer), brewsky (for beer), cold one (for beer)	Low dose: euphoria, relaxation, decreased inhibitions; higher doses, drowsiness, slurred speech, nausea, impaired memory, sexual dysfunction, emotional lability, loss of consciousness	Tremors, hallucinations, seizures, delirium tremens (with life-threatening increase in blood pressure and heart rate)
MDMA	Ecstasy, Adam, Eve, peace, lover's speed	Increased energy, euphoria, distortions in time, perception, and tactile experiences, feelings of empathy, hyperthermia	Loss of appetite, depression, attention deficits

Boards Boot Camp High-Yield Compendium

GHB	G, boy, liquid ecstasy, soap, scoop, liquid X	Sedation, memory loss, loss of coordination, possible coma	Insomnia, anxiety, sweating
Rohypnol (flunitrazepam)	R2, roach, roofies, roofinol, rope, rophies	Anterograde amnesia, sedation, muscle relaxation, confusion	Arrhythmias, anxiety
Salvia	Magic mint, Sally-D	Hallucinations, psychotomimetic episodes, feelings of being detached from self and environment (dissociation), uncontrollable laughter; after the peak effects, "afterglow" (prolonged pleasant state of mind)	None
Ketamine	Special K, vitamin K	Distorted perception, feelings of detachment from self and environment (dissociation), impaired attention and memory; at higher doses, dream-like states and hallucinations; at large doses, delirium and amnesia	Irritability, insomnia, intense depression
Anabolic steroids	Roids, juice, gym candy, pumpers	No intoxication – but chronic or recurrent use causes anger, "roid rage," violence, aggression, mood swings, paranoid jealousy, blood clots, acne, baldness, testicular atrophy, gynecomastia, infertility, and risk for prostate cancer	Mood swings, fatigue, lost libido and appetite, insomnia

LSD	Acid, blotter, microdot, cubes	Visual hallucinations, cross-over delusions (hear colors and see sounds), paranoid delusions, dilated pupils	None
Inhalants (e.g., paint thinner, glue, butane, aerosol propellants)	Poppers, snappers, whippets	Loss of inhibition, headache, slurred speech, loss of motor coordination	Excessive sweating, insomnia, hallucinations, aggressiveness, psychosis
Spice	K2, skunk, moon rocks	Elevated mood, altered perception, relaxation	Variable
Marijuana	Blunt, ganja, grass, herb, joint, bud, Mary Jane, pot, reefer, green, smoke, skunk, weed	Distorted perception, euphoria, impaired coordination, cognitive dysfunction, increased appetite; higher dose or chronic use: panic attacks, psychosis	Irritability, insomnia, decreased appetite, anxiety
Nicotine	Cigarettes, cigars, chew, snuff	Relaxation, increased blood pressure and heart rate	Irritability, increased appetite, attention deficits, sleep disturbance
Amphetamines	Bennies, black beauties, hearts, speed, truck drivers, uppers	Appetite suppression, insomnia, improved attention and focus, +/- euphoria (if snorted or injected)	Fatigue, depression, sleep disturbance
Substituted cathinones (e.g., mephedrone, methylone, MDPV)	Bath salts (other names include red dove, blue silk, zoom, bloom, vanilla sky, cloud nine)	Hallucinations, extreme paranoia, delusions, extreme agitation, extreme violence, malignant hypertension, palpitations, loss of pain sensation, dilated pupils	Fatigue, depression, decreased appetite, sleep disturbance

Boards Boot Camp High-Yield Compendium

Phencyclidine	Angel dust, PCP, hog, boat	Low dose: Euphoria, less inhibition Higher dose: anxiety, violence, lack of sensation Large dose: paranoia, auditory hallucinations Massive dose: kidney failure, arrhythmia, seizures, death	Diarrhea, chills, tremors, seizures, hallucinations; long-term withdrawal effects (e.g., long after drug cessation) include depression, cognitive impairment, and memory loss
Khat	Arabian tea, gat	Euphoria, elation, feelings of increased alertness and awareness, manic behavior, dilated pupils, loss of appetite	Nightmares, tremor
Opioids, opiates, narcotics	Street names for heroin: smack, horse, brown sugar, junk, skag, skunk	Euphoria, apathy, respiratory depression, pinpoint pupils	Nausea, vomiting, sweating, fever, muscle aches
Benzodiazepines	Benzos, chill pill, downers, roach	Sedation	Anxiety, insomnia, irritability

Section 100.4   <u>Child Abuse</u>

Abuse can be physical, emotional, sexual, or that of neglect. Most abuse occurs within the family unit, or people known to the family.

<u>PHYSICAL ABUSE</u>
Infants and young children are at higher risk
Sickly or disabled children are at the highest risk
Premature or low birth weight infants are at particular risk
Females are the more common abuser
Risk factors for physical abuse include guardian/parent drug abuse,
guardian/parent history of physical abuse when a child, poverty

Findings that Raise Concern for Physical Abuse: ANY injury (burn, bruise, fracture, head injury, abdominal injury) that cannot be explained; injuries that are particularly concerning are those to the back or the plantar foot, and those that have clearly demarcated edges.

A history of multiple injuries should also raise red flags!

Also, studies show that children are 100 times more often murdered by a non-biological parent (step-parent, boyfriend/girlfriend) than the biological parent

EMOTIONAL ABUSE

This is also known as psychological or mental abuse

It is the most common type of child abuse in the US

Emotional abuse can include loud yelling, rude or disrespectful behavior, harsh criticism, name-calling, ridicule, torture or killing of a pet, destruction of toys or other personal belongings, "silent treatment," things said or done to humiliate the child

Findings that Raise Concern: fearful behavior, nightmares, depression, shyness

SEXUAL ABUSE

Pre-adolescents and adolescents are at highest risk

Males are usually (but not always!) the abuser

The abuser is usually known to the victim

Risk factors for sexual abuse include guardian/parent drug abuse and single parent homes

Findings that Raise Concern: genital pain or bleeding, sexually transmitted disease, nocturnal enuresis or encopresis, extreme sexual behavior that is inappropriate for the child's age

In the US, up to 1 in 4 women and up to 1 in 7 men were sexually abused as children.

<u>NEGLECT</u>
Children born from unintended pregnancies are at the highest risk
Neglect is the failure to meet the child's basic needs
Neglect can be physical, educational, emotional, or medical
It is the second-most common type of abuse in the US, and the #1 type that is formally reported to officials
Physical neglect involves not providing the necessities of life, such as food and clothing.
Educational neglect involves failing to provide educational or enriching experiences for the child
Emotional neglect includes not providing emotional support or assurance, or even, in some cases, acknowledgement of presence (e.g., ignored)
Medical neglect involves failing to provide for the child's basic needs for maintenance of health
Risk factors include guardian/parent mental illness or drug abuse, domestic violence, and poverty

Section 101.0   <u>Sleep Stages</u>

Awake	fully awake	beta waves	>14 cycles/sec
	when in a quiet, resting state	alpha waves	8-13 waves/sec
Stage 1		"the head bob stage"	
		alpha waves	8-13 waves/sec
		theta waves	4-7 waves/sec
Stage 2 (about 45-50% of sleep)		theta waves 4-7 waves/sec	
		spindles (peaks of brain waves become higher and higher) 6-12 waves/sec	
		K-complexes (peaks that suddenly and drastically descend but then return to baseline; occur after spindles)	
Stage 3 (approx. 15-20% of sleep)		theta waves	4-7 waves/sec
		delta waves	0.5-4 waves/sec (comprise 20-50% of all waves in this stage)

Stage 4 (approx. 15-20% of sleep)	theta waves	4-7 waves/sec
	delta waves	0.5-4 waves/sec (comprise >50% of all waves in this stage)
	the most restful state and the deepest stage of sleep	
REM (approx. 20-25% of sleep)	beta waves	>14 cycles/sec (like awake!)
	Rapid eye movement, dreams	

Stages 1-4 are known as slow wave sleep (SWS) or NREM (non-REM sleep).

Stages 3 and 4 are the stages of night terrors, sleep talking, sleep walking (somnambulism), and enuresis.

Stages 3 and 4 shorten as the night progresses, becoming shorter and shorter with each repeat of the cycle.

Stages 3 and 4 are the most restful and restorative periods of sleep. That means that the most beneficial period of sleep is the beginning, since stages 3 and 4, and therefore restorative sleep, shorten as the night progresses. The best sleep is gained through naps that allow for at least one cycle of stages 3 and 4, which are the longest in the first cycle.

Stages 3 and 4 are the periods of the day in which the most restoration and replenishment to the immune system, and all immune system components, are made. Likewise, stages 3 and 4 are those periods of the day (both awake and asleep) in which the greatest amount of growth hormone is released; this permits for growth of children and for healing of injuries and illness in persons of all ages.

During REM, there is paralysis of skeletal muscles except for eyes, fingers and toes; there is increased BP and respiration rate, there is penis erection, and there are dreams and nightmares (these are the nightmares that are usually remembered).

REM is hypothesized, and supported through studies, to be critical to consolidation of memory for things experienced while awake; this is especially so for topics that require thought and synthesis. Those who take a test without a full night's sleep beforehand are statistically more likely to do poorly since they were not benefited by REM which puts all memory and knowledge in a form that is accessible and usable.

Boards Boot Camp High-Yield Compendium

When a person sleeps, they cycle through stage 1, then stage 2, then stage 3, then stage 4, then VERY rapidly reverse through stages 3, 2, then 1, to arrive quickly to REM sleep. Each cycle up to REM is about 90 minutes; then REM occurs. Therefore, each cycle lasts 100 minutes to 150 minutes, since REM varies. In the first cycle of the night, the first REM encountered is usually 10 minutes long. As the night progresses, each subsequent REM gets longer and longer, eventually reaching a maximum duration of about 1 hour/

All cycles repeat through-out the night.

For the most benefit from sleep, infants should get 16-18 hours of sleep/day, children should get 9-10 hours of sleep per day, teens should get 9 hours/day, and adults should get no less than 7-8 hours per day. Elderly adults require as much sleep as young adults. However, the elderly have shortened stages 3 and 4, making their sleep less beneficial, especially as the night wears on. Thus, the elderly would benefit much from naps during the day in order to gain several deep sleep stages over a 24 hours period (and, remember, the longest stages 3 and 4 that one will have will always be in the 1st cycle…so multiple short sleep periods in addition to regular night-time sleep is more beneficial to the elderly than one long sleep period at night).

MORVAN'S SYNDROME: An autoimmune disease that features anti-potassium channel antibodies. These individuals go without any sleep for months at a time. They have multiple physical and psychiatric issues as a result.

Section 102.0   PSYCHIATRY

Major Defense mechanisms

Regression = childish response to stress
Repression = suppression from awareness of any emotions and memories experienced as painful
Denial =   ignoring an undesired situation and behaving as if it does not exist although person knows full well it does exist
Rationalization = substituting an acceptable motive for attitudes and behavior that really have an unacceptable motive
Splitting =   seeing all things and people as either all good or all bad (so you are either their very, very good friend or their mortal enemy)
Projection =   attributing to others unwanted ideas or feelings that one is actually experiencing within oneself

Section 102.1   NEUROTRANSMITTERS

Pathology	**Neurotransmitter Anomaly**
Schizophrenia	increased dopamine
Other Psychoses	increased dopamine
Depression	decreased norepinephrine, serotonin, dopamine
Alzheimer's	decreased acetylcholine
Anxiety	decreased GABA
Low Pain Threshold	decreased serotonin

Section 102.2   PERSONALITY DISORDERS

Personality Types ←—————————→ Personality Disorders
(normal)   (pathologic)

Normal individuals are thought to have a mixture of all the personality types without a preponderance of any one type.

Those persons with personality disorders ("Axis II Psychiatric Disorders") have one personality style as their preponderant or sole personality type.

Schizotypal	the type to wear unmatched shoes or a coat in summer, have bizarre behavior, abnormal perception of reality → may become schizophrenic
Schizoid	wants no close relationships (the hermit)
Avoidant	wants close relationships but afraid to form them
Borderline	INTENSE but unstable relationships, self-damaging (often cut arms to relieve stress), suicidal and sometimes homicidal behavior is common, may be somewhat paranoid, undertakes a splitting defense mechanism frequently
Paranoid	perpetually distrusts others and is suspicious of others' motives
Antisocial	pervasively disregards and violates the rights of others; has no ability to feel empathy for man or beast and has little to no sympathetic response to normally dangerous or frightening things that would prevent an average person from engaging in certain activities – the combination of those two elements allows for actions against people and animals that are actions typically condemned by society
Histrionic	excessively emotional; all behavior geared towards attention seeking – tend to be very gregarious and sexually promiscuous
Narcissistic	has a pervasive fantasy or behavior consistent with a sense of grandiosity, a need for admiration, and a lack of empathy
Dependent	needs to be taken care of and, as a result, exhibits submissive and clinging behavior

| **Obsessive-Compulsive** | exhibits a preoccupation with perfectionism, orderliness, and control over self and others, at the expense of flexibility, efficiency, and open-mindedness. |

Section 102.3   SOMATOFORM DISORDERS

This is a group of disorders characterized by physical complaints that occur in absence of identifiable physical pathology or, as is more common, occur in association with an exaggeration of signs and symptoms not consistent with the degree of pathology present.

The Type of Somatoform Disorders include:
1) Somatization Disorder
2) Conversion Disorder
3) Hypochondriasis
4) Body Dysmorphic Disorder

Somatization Disorder
(Briquet's Syndrome)
Lasts many years, usually starting before age 30
Always involves pain and must, at least, involve:
4 pain complaints (different ones)
2 GI complaints
1 sexual complaint (other than pain)
1 pseudoneurologic complaint (e.g., neurologic problems with no identifiable cause or reason: blindness, deafness, feeling of lump in throat, urinary retention, etc)

Conversion Disorder

always neuro complaints

Lasts briefly (days, weeks)
Patient is NOT faking!
NO pain is involved – patient only has pseudoneurologic complaints, e.g. blindness (with no physical cause and no findings on funduscopic examination)
Symptoms occur in synchrony with psychological factors (stress, anxiety, etc.)

Hypochondriasis

Preoccupation with fears or concerns over having serious disease, based upon person's exaggerated misinterpretation of symptoms
Preoccupation persists despite favorable medical evaluation, and persists for > 6 months

Body Dysmorphic Disorder

Preoccupation with an imagined bodily defect or deficit affecting one's appearance, or preoccupation with an exaggerated concern over a slight physical imperfection
Most common preoccupations involve facial features, hair, breasts, size and shape of genitalia – and patients often spend hours each day gazing in a mirror at that body part

Section 102.4   ANXIETY DISORDERS

Panic Disorder

recurrent, unexpected panic attacks (during panic attacks, patients will experience intense fear or psychological discomfort along with at least 4 of the following symptoms: palpitations, sweating, paresthesias, fear of losing control, dizziness, nausea, chest pain or tightness, trembling, shortness of breath, choking sensation)
Tx: benzodiazepines for acute problems, but chronically should be treated with an SSRI or a TCA

Phobic Disorder a marked, excessive fear triggered by the presence or anticipation of a certain object or situation; exposure to that object or situation provokes intense anxiety

Tx: psychotherapy is the treatment of choice; benzodiazepines or beta-blockers can be used for specific, isolated events

Generalized Anxiety Disorder

excessive worry and apprehensive anticipation (>6 months) over multiple events, plans, objects; the so-called "worry wart"

more common in females; starts in early adulthood

Tx: psychotherapy + benzodiazepines

Section 102.5   **POST-TRAUMATIC STRESS DISORDER**

- Is also a type of anxiety disorder!
- Person has been exposed to a horrific traumatic event (e.g., war, assault, rape, witnessing trauma, etc.)
- The event is persistently re-experienced through intrusive recollections, and/or recurrent dreams, and/or "reliving" the sensations or feelings of the event; or patient experiences intense physical or psychological distress when exposed to something resembling the event

- Experience hyperarousal with at least 2 of the following: 1) exaggerated startle response, 2) insomnia, 3) outbursts of anger, 4) hypervigilance, 5) decreased concentration and focus.
- Treatment of choice is psychotherapy

Section 102.6   MOOD DISORDERS

Major Depressive Disorder
❖ Symptoms have to be present for at least 2 weeks
❖ Feelings of sadness, hopelessness, and worthlessness are the "triad"
❖ Tx: 1st line – SSRIs; 2nd line- TCAs or SNRIs; 3rd line – MAOIs; all with or without psychotherapy
❖ For the diagnosis, a patient must have at least 5 of the following problems, which MUST include depressed mood or anhedonia as one of the 5 criteria:

SIGECAPS

1) recurrent thoughts of suicide
2) **depressed mood** (sad)
3) **anhedonia** (loss of interest in things once enjoyed)
4) decreased focus or concentration skills
5) significant change in body weight (decreased weight without dieting or increased weight)
6) insomnia or hypersomnia
7) fatigue
8) feelings of worthlessness or excessive guilt
9) psychomotor agitation (one example would be "fidgetiness")

Boards Boot Camp High-Yield Compendium

Dysthymic Disorder
* ❖ Symptoms must be present for at least 2 years
* ❖ Depressed mood (observed by patient OR others) with 2 or more of the following:
    1) Appetite changes
    2) Insomnia or hypersomnia
    3) Low energy
    4) Low self-esteem
    5) Poor concentration
* ❖ Does not meet criteria for MDD (need 5)
* ❖ Tx: TCAs, MAOIs, SNRIs, or SSRIs, plus psychotherapy

Bipolar Disorder
* ❖ There are 2 types:

BIPOLAR I DISORDER
Individual episodes of mania preceded or followed by episodes of depression

BIPOLAR II DISORDER
Individual episodes of hypomania preceded or followed by episodes of depression

Mania features any three or more of the following, to the extent of being harmful to self or others:

DIG FAST

1) feelings of grandiosity
2) hedonistic activities – often become promiscuous, disinhibited
3) hyposomnia – may not sleep at all
4) psychomotor agitation, or excessive goal-directed activities – can become frenzied
5) pressured speech
6) racing thoughts
7) decreased focus

Hypomania is a lesser version of mania in that the symptoms are much less severe and typically not socially impairing, and are NOT taken to the extent of being dangerous to self or others. In fact, these persons can often be very productive, very efficient, and extremely goal-oriented.

Treatment: Maintenance treatment drug of choice is lithium. Common alternatives are valproic acid and carbamazepine. Monotherapy is discouraged. Instead, the standard of treatment is to use two mood stabilizers together or to use one mood stabilizer medication with an atypical antipsychotic.

Ebstein anomaly

605

Section 102.7 PSYCHOTIC DISORDERS

Psychosis is marked by hallucinations and delusions. It is treated with anti-psychotic medications; the atypical anti-psychotics are preferred (the drug of choice is risperidone)

Psychotic Disorder Due to a General Medical Condition
❖ Psychosis that is due to a medical disorder; some medical disorders that can cause psychosis are:

Brain tumor
Wilson's disease   Copper   Flesh kieur nyp
CVA
SLE
Variant Creutzfeld-Jakob Disease   "mad cow"
Porphyria   heme
Vitamin B12 deficiency
Pellagra   niacin B3
Korsakoff's Psychosis (vitamin B1 deficiency)   thiamine
Neurosyphilis   trepomann pallidn
Alzheimer's Disease   ↓ Ach
Huntington's Disease   CAt repeat
Lead Poisoning
HIV Dementia
Herpes encephalitis

Psychotic Disorder due to Drugs

Drug examples that can cause psychosis include:

LSD

Marijuana

Methamphetamine

dilated pupil ↑symp

Cocaine – risk for psychosis increases with continued use (a process known as "reverse tolerance")

Ketamine

Salvia – a significant growing problem in the US and it is legal in many states

Dextramethorphan

Ecstasy (MDMA) – also causes neuronal atrophy and death, eventually producing the "swiss cheese" brain

Brief Psychotic Disorder

❖ Psychosis for at least 1 day, but < 1 month
❖ Tends to follow an extremely traumatizing event

Folie a Deux

❖ "shared psychotic disorder"
❖ A delusion develops in a person (who usually is in a submissive or dependent position) who has a close personal relationship with another person who already has delusions as part of a psychotic illness

Delusional Disorder

❖ Non-bizarre (e.g., believable) delusions that last for at least 1 month; delusions can include beliefs (that are unfounded) that one is being followed, or infected, or poisoned, or that one is very powerful, or all-knowing, etc.

Schizoaffective Disorder

❖ Symptoms of schizophrenia, + mood disorder (e.g., major depressive disorder)

❖ The disturbance is not due to drugs or a general medical conditions

❖ Symptoms must be present for > 6 months for the diagnosis

❖ The psychosis has to be present at some time for at least 2 weeks WITHOUT any mood symptoms (otherwise, instead of schizoaffective disorder with the primary disturbance being psychosis, it is considered to be a mood disorder with psychotic features - e.g., it is not schizoaffective disorder).

Schizophreniform Disorder

❖ Symptoms for at least 1 month, but < 6 months

❖ Symptoms are those of schizophrenia

❖ NOT due to drugs or a general medical condition

Schizophrenia

* Symptoms for 6 months or more
* Must include at least 2 of the following:
    1) delusions
    2) hallucinations
    3) disorganized speech
    4) disorganized behavior
    5) negative symptoms (flattened affect, alogia, etc.)
* NOT due to drugs or a general medical conditions

Facts about Schizophrenia and Related Disorders

* Schizophrenia (and schizophreniform and schizoaffective disorder) as well as schizotypal personality disorder and schizoid personality disorder are all considered to be related to one another, and to be expressions of different but related disorders on the same continuum of pathology
* These disorders tend to run in families (e.g., one family member might have schizophrenia, while another may have schizotypal disorder, and so forth)
* Most with these disorders demonstrate certain classic signs and symptoms in childhood such as auditory processing problems, poor social skills, and, sometimes blunting of affect (e.g., child is rarely seen to smile, etc.); mild brain atrophy is also evident
* Considered to be neurodevelopmental disorders

609

ANATOMY

Section 103.0   **Embryology and Fetal Development**

Section 103.1   **Germ Layer Development**

Week 1

Fertilization

Sperm penetrate corona radiata

Sperm bind to and penetrate the zona pellucida

Cell membranes of an ovum and a sperm fuse
(both nuclei are then contained in one
cell, and fuse to form a cell with a single
nucleus → the zygote)

Blastocyst Formation

Zygote divides once by mitosis to become a
blastula; at this stage the blastula has 2
blastomeres (cells)

Mitotic division continues, to get 4 blastomeres,
then 8, and so forth

The blastomeres on the outer layer of the "ball"
of cells form tight junctions with one
another, sealing in the cells in the inner
cell mass; the whole "ball" is known as a
morula

The morula secretes fluid between the cells,
forming a cavity of fluid (a blastocyst
cavity) within the morula; a morula with a
blastocyst cavity = a blastocyst

The inner cell mass of the
blastocyst = embryoblast

The outer cell mass of the
blastocyst = trophoblast

Zona pellucida degeneration

Occurs within 4 days after conception
(fertilization)

Implantation

Blastocyst implants (usually) on the superior aspect of the posterior wall (endometrial lining) by day 7 after conception (fertilization).

Trophoblast cells in the blastocyst divide and differentiate into cytotrophoblast and syncytiotrophoblast.

Week 2   Embryoblast proliferation and differentiation

Embryoblast differentiates into 2 layers of cells: epiblast and hypoblast.

Collectively, the hypoblast and the epiblast form a flat oval-shaped disk known as the bilaminar embryonic disk – it is the special shape the embryoblast assumes

Clefts form in the epiblast, and they coalesce to form a single cavity → the amniotic cavity (completely surrounded by epiblast cells)

Some hypoblast cells migrate to the trophoblast, specifically to the inner lining of the trophoblast (cytotrophoblast) → the result is a cavity lined by hypoblast cells (some with the embryoblast and some wrapping around on the inner side of the cytotrophoblast) → that cavity is known as the primitive yolk sac

Hypoblast cells become columnar in one area, and fuse with epiblast cells there to form a thick, circular area in the embryoblast midline; this is called the prochordal plate, and is the site of the future mouth.

Trophoblast proliferation and differentiation

Lacunae (lakes; openings) form within the syncytiotrophoblast (the most outer lining of the blastocyst)

Boards Boot Camp High-Yield Compendium

The syncytiotrophoblastic lacunae fill with maternal blood

The lacunae fuse together to form a lacunar network

Maternal blood flows into and out of the lacunar network → this is known as "uteroplacental circulation"

The cytotrophoblast proliferates and invades into the syncytiotrophoblast

The new, invaded cytotrophoblast cells produce groups of cells that bulge into the syncytiotrophoblast → these mounds of cells are the chorionic villi

EXTRAEMBRYONIC Mesoderm develops

Some epiblast cells migrate to the area surrounding the yolk sac, specifically to the area BETWEEN the inner lining of the yolk sac (hypoblast cells that previously migrated there → collectively known as extracoelomic membrane) and the cells just beneath the extracoelomic membrane (cytotrophoblast). So, between those 2 cell layers, some epiblast cells migrate. These epiblast cells in that area become the extraembryonic mesoderm.

Large spaces develop between the cells of the extraembryonic mesoderm → these spaces coalesce to form one large cavity known as the extraembryonic coelom

The extraembryonic mesoderm that is left lining the extraembryonic coelom on the inner side of the cavity (the side next to the extracoelomic membrane) is now termed extraembryonic visceral mesoderm; the extraembryonic mesoderm that is left lining the extraembryonic coelom on the outer side of the cavity (the side next to the cytotrophoblast) is now termed the extraembryonic somatic mesoderm. NOTE: Extraembryonic mesoderm is not the mesoderm of the embryo, and does not form organs – its only role is that of placental development

Extraembryonic somatic mesoderm + cytotrophoblast + syncytiotrophoblast = chorion

Now, the extraembryonic coelom is termed the chorionic cavity.

The embryoblast is suspended by a connecting stalk (comprised of mesoderm), dangling into the chorionic cavity.

Weeks 3–8   All major organ systems begin to develop

Gastrulation occurs at week 3

Epiblast cells proliferate in a streak down the top middle of the embryonic disk

This is the primitive streak; it consists of the primitive groove, primitive node, and primitive pit

In an area caudal to the primitive streak, some epiblast and hypoblast cells fuse in a small area; that becomes the cloacal membrane, the site of the future anus

Epiblast cells divide and migrate to form three layers from the original 1 layer of epiblast

Boards Boot Camp High-Yield Compendium

cells; those three cell layers are the endoderm (bottom or ventral layer), (intraembryonic) mesoderm (middle layer), and ectoderm (top or dorsal layer). NOTE: It is the INTRAEMBRYONIC mesoderm that is part of the embryo and that is involved with organ development.

Section 103.2 GERM LAYER DERIVATIVES

Ectoderm	Mesoderm	Endoderm
Epidermis of skin, hair	Muscle (smooth, cardiac, skeletal)	Hepatocytes
CNS		Epithelial lining of vagina, bladder, biliary tree, GI tract, respiratory tract, middle ear, most of urethra
Anterior pituitary	Connective tissue	
Retina, iris, optic nerve	Dermis of skin	
Lens	Bone and cartilage	
Posterior pituitary	Endothelial cells	
Myelin		
Melanocytes		

Neural tube is derived from ectoderm, and develops into CNS
Neural crest is derived from ectoderm, and develops into smooth muscle, peripheral nervous system, adrenal medulla, and melanocytes
Placodes are derived from ectoderm, and develop into the sensory organs
Somites are derived from mesoderm, and develop into skeletal muscle and the spine

Section 103.3   FETAL REMNANTS

Fetal Structure	Remnant in Adult
Foramen ovale	Fossa ovalis
Ductus arteriosus	Ligamentum arteriosum
Ductus venosus	Ligamentum venosum
Umbilical arteries	Medial umbilical ligaments
Urachus	Median umbilical ligament
Umbilical vein	Ligamentum teres hepatis (round ligament)
Yolk stalk (usually obliterates completely, but if it does not, will yield....	Meckel's diverticulum

Facts:
◊   The **foramen ovale** is also known as the **ostium secundum**, and allows blood to travel from the right atrium to the left atrium (it is one of 3 fetal shunts, and allows blood to bypass the non-functional fetal lungs)

◊   The **ductus arteriosus**, the another fetal shunt, connects the pulmonary artery to the aortic arch, allowing most of the blood from the right ventricle to bypass the non-functional fetal lungs.

◊   The **ductus venosus**, the third of three fetal shunts, shunts blood from the umbilical vein directly into the inferior vena cava, allowing oxygenated blood from the placenta to bypass the liver and get delivered to the systemic circulation (and brain) faster.

◊   The **umbilical cord** contains three vessels: 2 arteries and 1 vein

◊   The **umbilical arteries** serve to deliver <u>de-oxygenated</u> blood TO the placenta

◊   The **umbilical vein** serves to deliver <u>oxygenated</u> blood FROM the placenta

◊   The **yolk stalk**, also known as the **vitelline duct** or the **omphalomesenteric duct**, connects the yolk sac to the midgut, in the area of the future ileum

◊   The **urachus** connects the bladder with the **allantois** (the allantois helps the fetus exchange gases and handle liquid waste). Normally, the urachus degenerates to become the median umbilical ligament in the adult. If it, however, remains patent, it is termed a patent urachus; it causes a condition in which there is a hollow tube connecting the bladder and the umbilicus that facilitates urination through the umbilicus.

Meckel's diverticulum results from yolk stalk persistence. It occurs in 2% of people, is about 2 cm long, and occurs about 2 feet from the ileocecal junction (in the ileum). Remember: 2-2-2. If it becomes inflamed, it can imitate appendicitis, complete with right lower quadrant pain.

Section 104.0   EYE

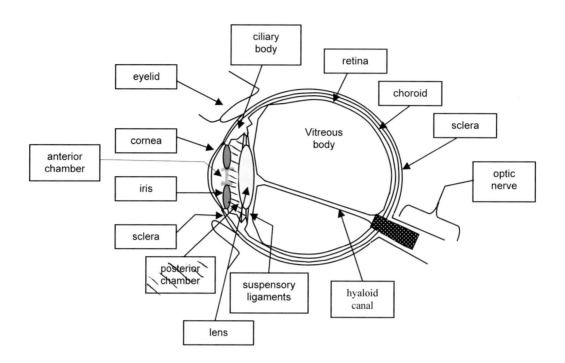

Cornea: transparent tissue over central area of anterior eye; is the area through which one can see into the eye to see the iris, the pupil, and the fundus.

Sclera: white, opaque fibrous coat (mostly collagen) that surrounds the entire eye except for the area occupied by the cornea; constitutes the "whites of the eyes." Provides structural support to eye.

Choroid: dark-brown tissue sandwiched between retina and sclera; easily lifted from sclera – but firmly attached to retina. Richly vascularized and provides nutrition to retina.

617

Ciliary body: is an extension of the choroid. Folds on its inner surface are termed the ciliary processes; they produce aqueous humor. Also contains the ciliary muscle which serves to, when contracted, allow relaxation of the suspensory ligaments (ciliary zonules) – this permits the lens to bulge or "plump up" for accommodation.

Iris: is an extension of the ciliary body. Heavily pigmented, and is what determines the "color" of our eyes. Has a central opening that is known as the pupil. Contains dilator pupillae muscles (for mydriasis) and sphincter pupillae muscles (for miosis).

> Specific eye color is determined by where the pigment is distributed in the iris. Blue eyes have pigment only on the posterior surface, brown eyes have it throughout, and green eyes have yet a different distribution.

Retina: internal to the choroid. Has two layers: the inner neural layer (innermost layer) and the outer pigmented layer. Most of retina is light sensitive, allowing for vision. It has a depression in the posterior part of the eye known as the optic disk – this is where optic fibers leave the eyeball to travel through the optic nerve and where retinal vessels enter.

Blind spot: the area of the optic disk (area where nerve fibers leave eyeball to travel through optic nerve) – has no photoreceptors so is insensitive to light.

Macula: properly termed the macula lutea, and is an oval yellow area that is lateral to the optic disk; within in it, in the center, is the fovea centralis. This is the area of most acute vision.

Posterior chamber: the chamber to which the ciliary processes release the aqueous humor they produce; located between the iris/ciliary body and the lens.

Anterior chamber: the area between the cornea and the iris/pupil. Aqueous humor arrives here, via travel through the pupil, from the posterior chamber.

Vitreous chamber: contains the vitreous body, and is located between the lens and the optic disk.

Aqueous humor: clear, watery fluid; produced by posterior chamber, delivered to anterior chamber through pupil, and exits anterior chamber via canals of Schlemm (canals that deliver the fluid from the most lateral aspects of the anterior chamber to the anterior ciliary vein of the scleral plexus).

Vitreous humor: transparent mass of jelly-like substance that is contained in the hyaloid (vitreous membrane); is located between the lens and retina.

Eyegrounds = fundus of the eye as seen with an ophthalmoscope

Fundus = the back of the eye, internally (where the retina and optic disk are)

The parts of the eye used for **refraction** (for sight):
Cornea
Aqueous humor
Lens
Vitreous body

Myopia: nearsightedness; eyeball is too long
Hyperopia: farsightedness; eyeball is too short
Presbyopia: old sight; lens lose its flexibility
Emmetropia: normal sight

Macular degeneration: Degeneration of macula; causes loss of central vision

Glaucoma: Increased aqueous humor causes increased intraocular tensions, resulting in "pressure" inside eyeball that ends up also being translated against the neural layer of retina; blindness can result.

Cataracts: Lens becomes opaque, preventing optimal visual acuity (everything appears cloudy). Recurrent or chronic hyperglycemia is a common cause → glucose enters lens and can easily diffuse out; but, if present chronically or recurrently, there is a higher chance that it will become sorbitol. Sorbitol cannot diffuse out again, but is osmotic ("draws" water with it). So, lens accumulates sorbitol and, as a consequence, bulges.

Section 104.1 Extraocular Muscles

Extraocular muscles are also known as extrinsic muscles of the eye. Their actions are noted below (which differ from "tests" of these muscles):

Superior rectus: makes pupil go up and slightly medially, and makes whole eyeball spin medially (no change in pupil position because of the spin, but a lateral eye lesion will look more superior as a result). Innervated by the oculomotor nerve (III).

Inferior rectus: makes pupil go down and slightly lateral, and makes whole eye ball spin laterally (no change in pupil position because of the spin, but a lateral eye lesion will look more inferior). Innervated by the oculomotor nerve (III).

Medial rectus: makes pupil move medially. Innervated by the oculomotor nerve (III).

Lateral rectus: makes pupil move laterally. Innervated by the abducens nerve (VI).   Abduct?

Superior oblique: moves pupil down and laterally; also makes eyeball spin medially (no change in pupil position because of the spin, but a lateral eye lesion will look more superior). Innervated by the trochlear nerve (IV).

Inferior oblique: moves pupil up and laterally; also makes eyeball spin laterally (no change in pupil position because of the spin, but a lateral eye lesion will look more inferior). Innervated by the oculomotor nerve (III).

Levator Palpebrae: raises upper eyelid. Innervated via the oculomotor nerve (III).

Section 105.0   NEUROANATOMY

The Basic Structures:

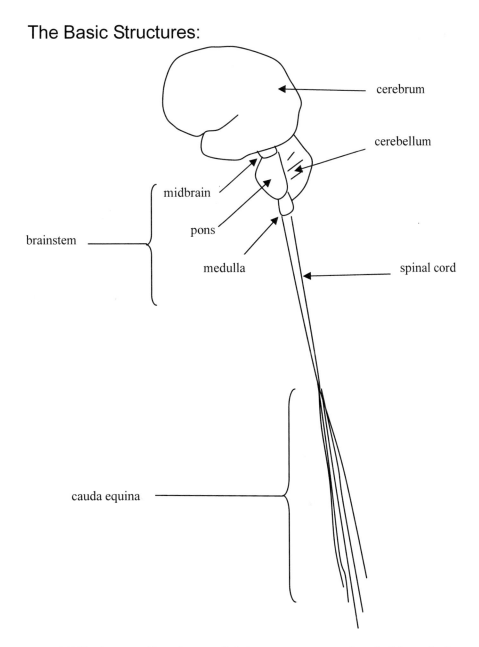

Section 105.1   Basics of Neuroanatomical Blood Supply

Common carotid artery
Common carotid divides to become internal and external carotid arteries. The internal carotid artery enters brain.

Internal carotid artery

Branches:

1st branch → **Ophthalmic artery** → travels through optic nerve
    Supplies retina
    Obstruction causes monocular blindness in the eye
    affected

Posterior communicating artery → joins posterior cerebral
    artery
        Supplies optic chiasm and tract, hypothalamus, ventral
            portion of thalamus
        A common site for berry aneurysms

Anterior choroidal artery
    Supplies many areas, including amygdala, globus pallidus

Anterior cerebral artery → courses along the medial side of
    hemisphere, in the cortex (outer layer of brain)
        Supplies the (medial) FRONTAL and PARIETAL LOBES →
            supplies the leg and foot areas of the motor and
            sensory cortex
        Gives off branches that supply the anterior portion of the
            internal capsule

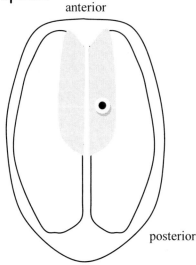

anterior

● A CVA located here
would cause motor
and/or sensory deficits
of the right lower
extremity

Cartoon Version of Head CT showing territory (in gray) **served by Anterior Cerebral Artery** – CVA in any part of that region would be associated with anterior cerebral artery pathology

RIGHT

posterior

Boards Boot Camp High-Yield Compendium

Anterior communicating artery → connects the 2 anterior
cerebral arteries
Is THE MOST COMMON site for berry aneurysms

Middle cerebral artery → courses along the lateral (outer)
side of the hemisphere, in the cortex (outer layer of
brain)
Supplies the (lateral) FRONTAL and PARIETAL LOBES →
supplies the trunk, arm, and face areas of the motor
and sensory cortex
Supplies Broca's and Wernicke's areas for speech
Gives off branches that supply the posterior limb of the
internal capsule

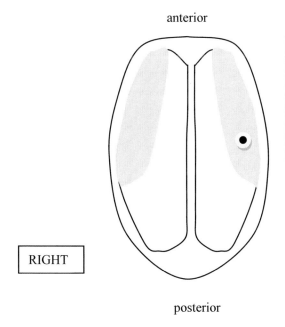

anterior

RIGHT

posterior

Cartoon Version of Head CT showing territory (in gray) **served by Middle Cerebral Artery** – CVA in any part of that region would be associated with ~~anterior~~ *middle* cerebral artery pathology

● A CVA located here would cause motor and/or sensory deficits of the right trunk, right arm, or left face; since it is in the left brain, it may also cause Broca's or Wernicke's aphasia

Vertebral artery
Represents a branch of the subclavian artery
The 2 vertebral arteries fuse to become the basilar artery
Branches of the vertebral artery are:

Anterior spinal artery

Posterior inferior cerebellar artery → gives rise to the
    posterior spinal artery
      Supplies the dorsolateral medulla and the inferior surface
        of the cerebellum

Basilar artery
Its branches include:

Pontine arteries
    Supply corticospinal tracts

Anterior inferior cerebellar artery → gives rise to the
    labyrinthine artery
      Supplies inferior cerebellar surface, + the trigeminal
        nucleus and tract, facial nucleus, vestibular nuclei,
        and cochlear nuclei + the spinothalamic tract of the
        pons

Superior cerebellar artery

Supplies the superior cerebellar surface + the lateral and rostral pons + the spinothalamic tract

Posterior cerebral artery

Is formed by the bifurcation of the basilar artery

Supplies the midbrain, the occipital lobe (and visual cortex), and inferior surface of the temporal lobes

Bottom-line: **Basilar Artery**, with its branches, serves the brainstem and cerebellum!

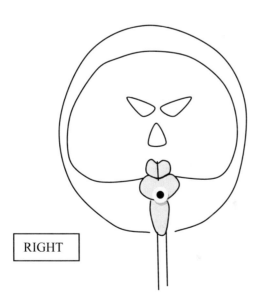

RIGHT

Cartoon Version of Head CT (coronal plane) **showing territory** (in gray) **served by branches of Basilar Artery** – CVA in any part of that region would be associated with pathology of the basilar artery or its branches

● A CVA located here (medial inferior pons) would cause weakness of lower left face, loss of left eye lateral gaze, ataxia, and right hemiparesis of the trunk and limbs, plus loss of right-sided proprioception and vibration sense (=Medial Inferior Pontine Syndrome)

Section 105.2 Cranial Nerves and Their Functions

CN1 Olfactory nerve Smell

CN2 Optic nerve Sight

CN3 Oculomotor nerve Eye movement – both the eyeball and the pupil (hence "oculo-MOTOR")

CN4 Trochlear nerve Eye movement (adduction) (the only cranial nerve that crosses over; thus damage to its nucleus causes contralateral eye movement effects)

CN5 Trigeminal nerve Sensation/pain

CN6 Abducens nerve Eye movement (abduction)

CN7 Facial nerve Facial movement, taste (anterior 2/3 of tongue)

CN8 Vestibulocochlear nerve Hearing, balance

CN9 Glossopharyngeal nerve Taste (poster 1/3 of tongue), swallowing, carotid body and sinus monitoring

CN10 Vagus nerve Taste (epiglottis), swallowing, palate movement, phonation, innervation of viscera of thoracic and abdominal cavity

CN11 Accessory nerve Turns head, lifts shoulders

CN12 Hypoglossal nerve Moves tongue (hence "glossal")

Section 105.2.1 The Facial Nerve

❖ Upper motor neuron damage (e.g., brain) to CN 7 causes only deficits in lower facial motor control.

❖ Lower motor neuron damage (e.g., facial nerve itself) causes the entire side of the face to lose motor control

Boards Boot Camp High-Yield Compendium

Innervation of Facial Muscles

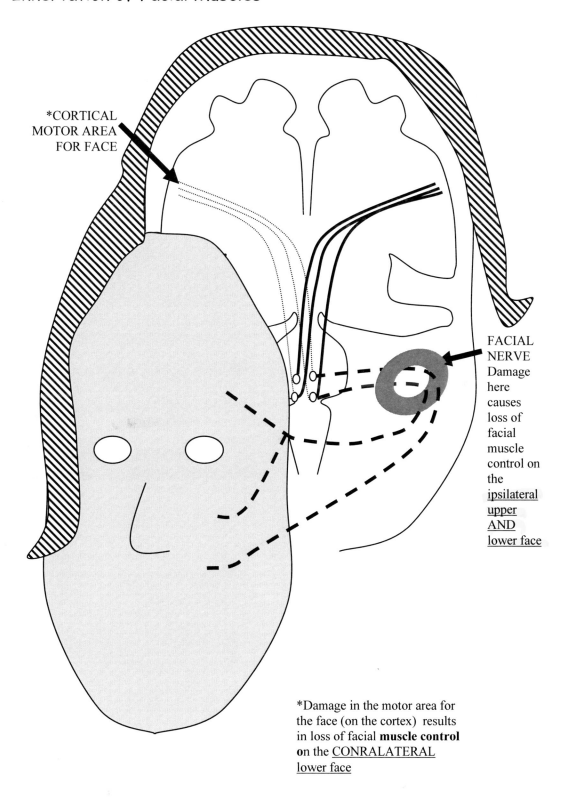

*CORTICAL
MOTOR AREA
FOR FACE

FACIAL
NERVE
Damage
here
causes
loss of
facial
muscle
control on
the
ipsilateral
upper
AND
lower face

*Damage in the motor area for
the face (on the cortex) results
in loss of facial **muscle control**
on the CONRALATERAL
lower face

Section 105.2.2   The Optic Nerve and Visual Field

To understand the visual fields and optical pathways, one must look at the following pathway diagram and interpret it as if you were looking from above, down onto the person's head. Alternatively, when interpreting the visual field defects (as depicted with double circles), you must pretend that you are looking THROUGH the patient's eyes, seeing or not seeing what they are seeing or not seeing. For instance, if ◐ ○ is depicted, it means the patient has full and normal visual field in the right eye, but loss of medial (nasal side) visual field in the left eye.

When an image (e.g., light) enters the eyes, images on the right side of the body enter the temporal side of the left retina (see below), as well as the nasal side of the right eye. Images on the left side of the body enter the eyes and hit the nasal side of the left retina and the temporal side of the right retina. Impulses are then sent from the retina to the optic nerve. Medial fibers of the optic nerve cross over to the other side of the brain at the optic chiasm. Lateral fibers of the optic nerve remain on the same side of the brain. All fibers then form the optic tract, after the optic chiasm. Eventually, the fibers split into "radiations," collectively known as the optic radiation. Some of those radiations travel in the parietal lobe, and the others travel in the temporal lobe. Those radiations are separated at this point into superior or inferior images. The parietal lobe radiations carry images projected onto the superior retina; images projected onto the superior retina are images of objects inferior to the patient's body. The temporal lobe radiations carry images projected onto the inferior retina; images projected onto the inferior retina are images of objects superior to the patient's body. Eventually, all fibers end at the calcarine fissure in the occipital lobe, specifically ending at the visual cortex. The center point of vision is handled by a part of the occiput that is supplied by an alternate arterial source, meaning that a central 5-10 degrees of sight is potentially spared in the event of occipital lobe damage. The loss of all other visual fields except for the center field is known as macular sparing. While the occiput is generally supplied by the posterior cerebral artery, there is evidence that the occipital pole is supplied instead by the middle cerebral artery (allowing for macular sparing).

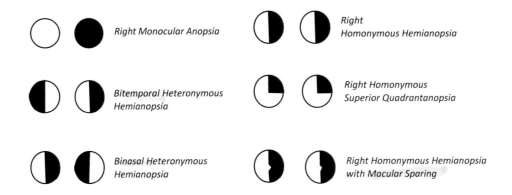

629

Visual Fields and Optical Pathways

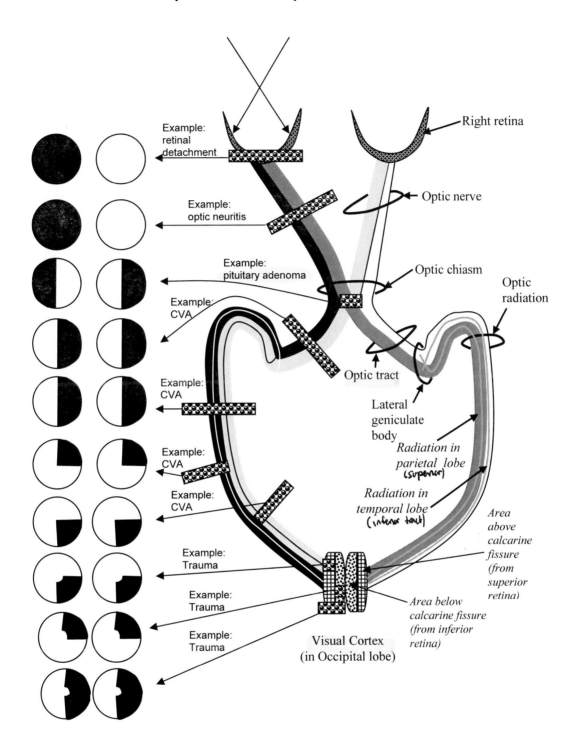

Example:
retinal
detachment

Example:
optic neuritis

Example:
pituitary adenoma

Example:
CVA

Example:
CVA

Example:
CVA

Example:
CVA

Example:
Trauma

Example:
Trauma

Example:
Trauma

Right retina

Optic nerve

Optic chiasm

Optic radiation

Optic tract

Lateral geniculate body

Radiation in parietal lobe (superior)

Radiation in temporal lobe (inferior tract)

Area above calcarine fissure (from superior retina)

Area below calcarine fissure (from inferior retina)

Visual Cortex
(in Occipital lobe)

Section 106.0 Brainstem Lesions

Brainstem = midbrain + pons + medulla

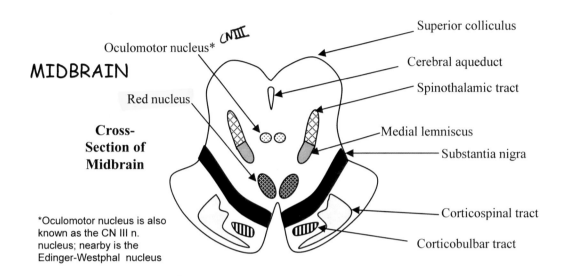

Oculomotor nucleus*   CN III

MIDBRAIN

Red nucleus

Cross-Section of Midbrain

Superior colliculus

Cerebral aqueduct

Spinothalamic tract

Medial lemniscus

Substantia nigra

Corticospinal tract

Corticobulbar tract

*Oculomotor nucleus is also known as the CN III n. nucleus; nearby is the Edinger-Westphal nucleus

MIDBRAIN

- ❖ damaged via vascular occlusion of the posterior cerebral artery (a branch of the basilar artery)
- ❖ damaged by hydrocephalus or pineal gland tumors
- ❖ damage to the dorsal midbrain results in damage to the superior colliculus and pretectal area (causes paralysis of upward and downward gaze, pupillary abnormalities, and loss of convergence) + damage to the cerebral aqueduct (yielding hydrocephalus); it is usually due to pinealomas

631

❖ damage to the medial midbrain causes Weber's syndrome; it results from occlusion of the branches of the posterior cerebral artery. It results in many deficits:

1) damage to oculomotor nerve roots (with paralysis of CN III-innervated extraocular muscles, yielding eye abduction and depression due to the unopposed action of CN VI and CN IV) └ *down & out*

2) damage to corticobulbar tracts, resulting in weakness of the ipsilateral lower face, tongue, and palate (since nerve fibers from CN VII, XII, and X are conveyed via the corticobulbar tract here)

3) damage to the corticospinal tract, resulting in contralateral hemiparesis of the entire trunk and extremities *above medulla decussation*

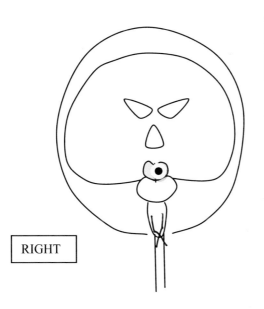

RIGHT

Cartoon Version of Head CT (coronal plane) **showing Midbrain** (in gray)

● A CVA located here (medial midbrain) would cause left eye abduction and depression, left-sided lower face, tongue, and palate weakness, and right-sided hemiparesis of the trunk and extremities (=**Weber's Syndrome**)

❖ damage to the paramedian midbrain results from occlusion of or hemorrhage from the posterior cerebral artery; it causes many deficits:

1) damage to oculomotor (CN III) nerve roots

2) damage to the red nucleus and dentarubrothalamic tract, resulting in intention tremor with contralateral cerebellar dystaxia

3) damage to the medial lemniscus, resulting in contralateral loss of vibration sense and proprioception

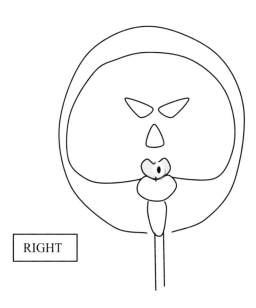

Cartoon Version of Head CT (coronal plane) **showing Midbrain** (in gray)

● A CVA located here (paramedian midbrain) would cause left eye abduction and depression, intention tremor, and right-sided loss of vibration sense and proprioception

RIGHT

633

PONS

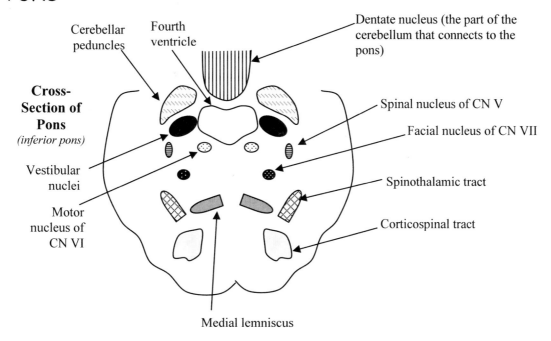

Cross-Section of Pons
(inferior pons)

Cerebellar peduncles

Fourth ventricle

Dentate nucleus (the part of the cerebellum that connects to the pons)

Spinal nucleus of CN V

Facial nucleus of CN VII

Spinothalamic tract

Corticospinal tract

Vestibular nuclei

Motor nucleus of CN VI

Medial lemniscus

❖ lesions result from occlusion of the basilar artery or any of its branches (anterior inferior cerebellar artery, transverse pontine arteries, and superior cerebellar artery)

❖ Medial inferior pontine syndrome results from occlusion of the paramedian branches of the basilar artery; the following deficits may occur:

1) damage to abducens (CN VI) nerve roots, resulting in loss of lateral rectus muscle function

2) damage to the base of the pons, resulting in ipsilateral ataxia and limb movement pathology

3) damage to the corticobulbar tracts, resulting in weakness of the lower face (since CN VII fibers are conducted here)]

4) damage to the corticospinal tracts, resulting in contralateral hemiparesis of the trunk and limbs

5) damage to the medial lemniscus, resulting in contralateral loss of proprioception and vibration sense

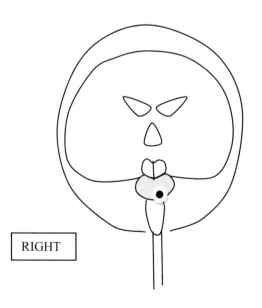

Cartoon Version of Head CT (coronal plane) **showing Pons** (in gray)

RIGHT

● A CVA located here (medial inferior pons) would cause loss of left eye lateral gaze, ataxia, weakness of left lower face, right-sided hemiparesis of trunk and limbs, and right-sided loss of proprioception and vibration sense (=**Medial Inferior Pontine Syndrome**)

❖ Lateral inferior pontine syndrome (AICA Syndrome) results from occlusion of the anterior inferior cerebellar artery; the following deficits may occur:

1) damage to the facial nucleus and nerve fibers (CN VII), resulting in ipsilateral facial muscle paralysis (lower face), loss of taste on the anterior 2/3 of tongue, and loss of corneal and stapedius reflexes.

2) damage to the cochlear nuclei and nerve fibers (CN VIII), resulting in unilateral nerve deafness

3) damage to the vestibular nuclei and nerve fibers (CN VIII), resulting in nystagmus, nausea, and vertigo

4) damage to the spinal trigeminal nucleus and tract (CN V), resulting in ipsilateral loss of facial pain and temperature sensation

5) damage to the middle and inferior cerebellar peduncles, resulting in ipsilateral dystaxia

6) damage to the spinothalamic tracts, resulting in contralateral pain and temperature sensation loss from the trunk and limbs

7) damage to the sympathetic tract, resulting in ipsilateral Horner's syndrome

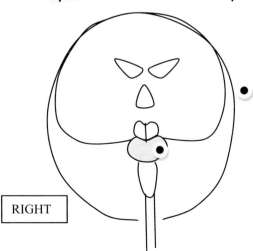

Cartoon Version of Head CT (coronal plane) showing Pons (in gray)

A CVA located here (lateral inferior pons) would cause left lower face paralysis, corneal reflex loss, and taste loss on anterior 2/3 of tongue, left-sided nerve deafness, nystagmus, nausea, vertigo, loss of left-sided facial pain and temperature sensation, dystaxia, loss of right-sided pain and temperature sensation of trunk and limbs, and left-sided Horner's syndrome (=**AICA SYNDROME**)

RIGHT

❖ Lateral midpontine syndrome results from obstruction of a branch off of the basilar artery; multiple deficits may occur:

1) damage to the trigeminal nuclei and nerve root (CN V) – motor and sensory – to result in paralysis of muscles of mastication, loss of corneal reflex, deviation of jaw to side of lesion (due to unopposed action of contralateral lateral pterygoid muscle), and ipsilateral loss of facial sense of pain, temperature, touch.

2) damage to middle cerebellar peduncle, resulting in dystaxia

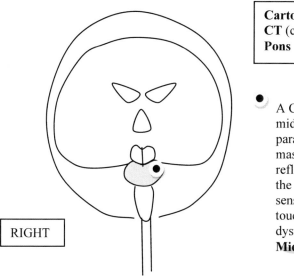

RIGHT

Cartoon Version of Head CT (coronal plane) **showing Pons** (in gray)

● A CVA located here (lateral middle pons) would cause paralysis of left muscles of mastication, loss of corneal reflex, deviation of the jaw to the left, loss of left-sided facial sense of pain, temperature, and touch, and would cause dystaxia (=**Lateral Midpontine Syndrome**)

637

❖ Lateral superior pontine syndrome results from obstruction of the superior cerebellar artery; it may result in multiple deficits:

1) damage to the superior and middle cerebellar peduncles, resulting in limb and trunk dystaxia

2) damage to the medial lemniscus, resulting in contralateral loss of proprioception and vibration sense

3) damage to the sympathetic tract, resulting in Horner's syndrome

4) damage to the spinothalamic tracts, resulting in contralateral loss of pain and temperature sense of the trunk + limbs; there is also ipsilateral facial loss of pain and temperature

5) damage to the dentate nucleus, resulting in dystaxia and intention tremor

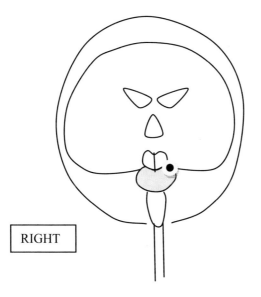

RIGHT

Cartoon Version of Head CT (coronal plane) **showing Pons** (in gray)

● A CVA located here (lateral superior pons) would cause limb and trunk dystaxia, right-sided loss of proprioception and vibration sense, left-sided Horner's syndrome, right-sided loss of pain and temperature sense of the trunk and limbs, left-sided loss of facial sense of pain and temperature, and intention tremor (=**Lateral Superior Pontine Syndrome**)

❖ Locked-in Syndrome (pseudo coma) is caused by central pontine myelinolysis (which is, itself, caused by correcting a hyponatremic patient's serum Na levels too quickly) or any cause that results in complete infarction or loss of function of the entire base of the pons; all motor function is lost except for the ability to blink or move eyes vertically

MEDULLA

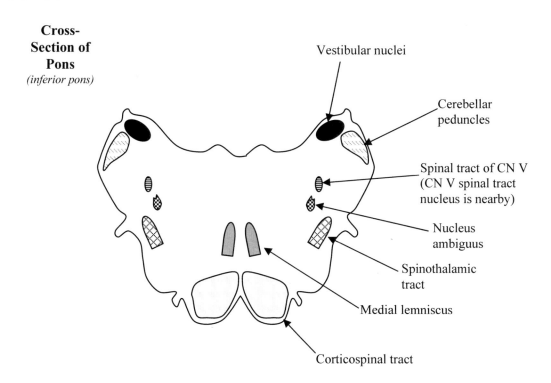

Cross-Section of Pons
(inferior pons)

Vestibular nuclei

Cerebellar peduncles

Spinal tract of CN V (CN V spinal tract nucleus is nearby)

Nucleus ambiguus

Spinothalamic tract

Medial lemniscus

Corticospinal tract

❖ Lesions of the medulla result from obstruction of the vertebral artery or any of its branches (anterior spinal artery or posterior inferior cerebellar artery)

❖ Medial medullary syndrome is damage to the medial medulla, and results from occlusion of the anterior spinal artery. Defects may include:

1) damage to the hypoglossal nerve roots (CN XII), resulting in ipsilateral flaccid paralysis of the tongue
2) damage to the medial lemniscus, resulting in contralateral loss of proprioception and vibration sense
3) damage to the corticospinal tract, resulting in contralateral hemiparesis of the trunk and limbs

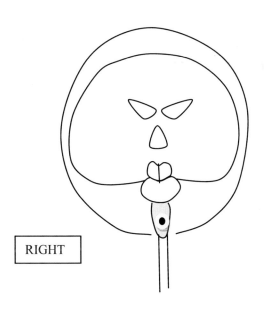

RIGHT

Cartoon Version of Head CT (coronal plane) **showing Medulla** (in gray)

● A CVA located here (medial medulla) would cause left-sided tongue paralysis, right-sided loss of proprioception and vibration sense, and right-sided hemiparesis of the trunk and limbs (= **Medial Medullary Syndrome**)

❖ Lateral medullary syndrome (PICA syndrome; Wallenberg's syndrome) involves damage to the lateral medulla. It is caused by obstruction of the vertebral or its branch, the posterior inferior cerebellar artery. Multiple deficits may occur:

1) damage to the inferior cerebellar peduncle, resulting in dystaxia, dysmetria
2) damage to the vestibular nuclei (CN VIII), resulting in nystagmus, vertigo, and nausea
3) damage to the nucleus ambiguus of CN IX, X, and XI, resulting in ipsilateral loss of the gag reflex, dysphagia, and hoarseness
4) damage to the sympathetic tract, resulting in Horner's syndrome
5) damage to the spinal trigeminal nucleus and tract, resulting in ipsilateral loss of facial pain and temperature sensation
6) damage to the glossopharyngeal nerve roots (CN IX), resulting in loss of gag reflex
7) damage to the vagal nerve roots (CN X), resulting in loss of gag reflex, dysphagia, and hoarseness
8) damage to the spinothalamic tracts, resulting in contralateral loss of pain and temperature sensation in the trunk and limbs

Boards Boot Camp High-Yield Compendium

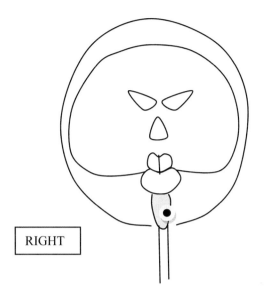

RIGHT

Cartoon Version of Head CT (coronal plane) **showing Medulla** (in gray)

- A CVA located here (lateral medulla) would cause dystaxia, dysmetria, nystagmus, vertigo, nausea, left-sided loss of gag reflex, and would cause dysphagia, hoarseness, left-sided Horner's syndrome, left-sided loss of facial pain and temperature sensation, right-sided loss of pain and temperature sensation in the trunk and limbs (= **PICA Syndrome**, also known as **Wallenberg's Syndrome**)

Section 107.0 Important Skull Holes

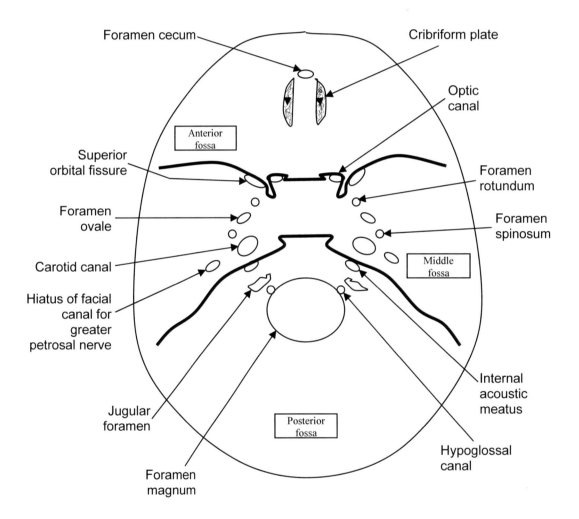

Skull Base: Interior View

Boards Boot Camp High-Yield Compendium

The Foramina and Other Important Openings of the Skull Base

Opening	Contents
Cribriform plate	Olfactory nerve fibers
Foramen cecum	Origin of superior sagittal venous sinus
Optic canal	Optic nerve and ophthalmic artery
Superior orbital fissure	Cranial nerves III, IV, VI, and cranial nerve V (ophthalmic branch), ophthalmic veins, sympathetic nerves
Foramen rotundum	Maxillary nerve √₂
Foramen ovale	Mandibular nerve and accessory meningeal artery V³
Foramen spinosum	Middle meningeal artery
Carotid canal	Carotid artery and sympathetic nerves
Hiatus for greater petrosal nerve	Greater petrosal nerve and petrosal branch of middle meningeal artery
Internal auditory meatus	Cranial nerve VII, VIII and internal auditory artery
Jugular foramen	Inferior petrosal and transverse sinuses, cranial nerves IX, X, and XI, and meningeal branches of the occipital and ascending pharyngeal arteries
Hypoglossal canal	Cranial nerve XII and meningeal branch of ascending pharyngeal artery
Foramen magnum	Spinal cord, vertebral arteries, anterior and posterior spinal arteries, and accessory nerve

Section 108.0 CLINICAL NEUROANATOMY

Spinal Cord Tracts

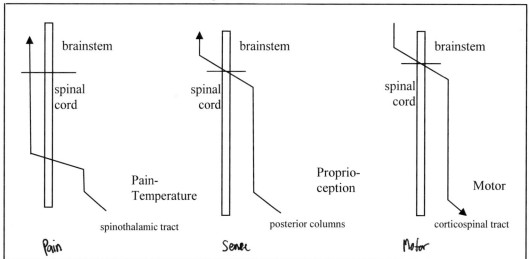

1. A patient status post motor vehicle accident is brought by EMS to the emergency department. There is spastic paralysis and loss of all sensory ability beginning near the level of the umbilicus and continuing all the way down the body bilaterally. There is increased patellar and Achilles deep tendon reflexes bilaterally.
    What occurred? UMN Complete transection of the spinal cord at T10

2. A patient is brought to the emergency room following a severe assault. There is paralysis beginning at the level of the umbilicus on the right side of the body. There is also decreased proprioception on the right side of the body in the same areas where there is paralysis. Achilles and patellar reflexes are 4/4 on the right and 2/4 on the left. On the left side of the body, there is decreased pain and temperature from a level about an inch below the umbilicus that extends all the way down the rest of the left side of the body.
    What occurred? Hemitransection of the right spinal cord at T10

3. A patient presents with complaints of "not being able to feel things like normal" throughout both his arms and across his shoulders, upper chest, and upper back. Examination reveals a patient with decreased light touch, proprioception, pain, and temperature sensation in a cape-like distribution over his upper body.
    What is the pathology? Syringomyelia

645

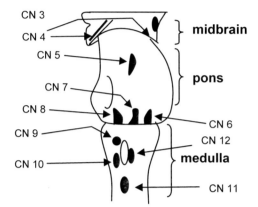

CN 3
CN 4
CN 5
CN 7
CN 8
CN 9
CN 10
} midbrain
} pons
CN 6
CN 12
} medulla
CN 11

THE BRAINSTEM

4.   A patient presents with paralysis of the entire left side of his body
       exclusive of the head and face. He also has tongue weakness allowing
       the tongue to deviate to the right. On examination, all left-sided deep
       tendon reflexes are increased, but perception of pain and temperature
       is intact. There is loss of proprioception on the left side of the body.
       Where is the lesion? right medulla

5.   A patient presents with severe weakness of the entire left side of the
       body, with the exception of the upper left face. DTRs on the left side of
       the body are increased, as well. He also has right facial anesthesia of the
       entire face, plus right masseter muscle weakness.
       Where is the lesion? right pons

6.   A patient presents with complaints of spastic paralysis of the entire right
       body except for the head. Triceps, biceps, patellar, and Achilles reflexes
       are 4/4 on the right and 2/4 on the left. He also has left facial weakness
       and is incapable of fully abducting the left eye.
       Where is the lesion? left pons (in caudal area)

7.   A patient presents with spastic paralysis of the entire left side of the body,
       with the exception of the left face. He also has difficulty adducting the
       right eye. On exam, there is right ptosis with a right dilated pupil. All
       DTRs on left extremities measure 4/4. Muscle strength is 0/5 on the left
       side of the body. There is no sensory loss.
       Where is the lesion? right midbrain
       What if the problems were all sensory related (decreased sensory
       ability) instead of spastic motor problem, but kept the decreased
       right eye adduction ability, continued the ptosis, and a right dilated
       pupil?   right midbrain

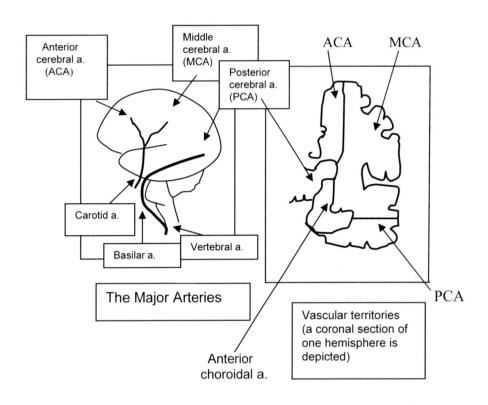

Anterior
cerebral a.
(ACA)

Middle
cerebral a.
(MCA)

Posterior
cerebral a.
(PCA)

Carotid a.

Basilar a.

Vertebral a.

The Major Arteries

Anterior
choroidal a.

ACA   MCA

PCA

Vascular territories
(a coronal section of
one hemisphere is
depicted)

Sensory Distribution over the Cortex
(one hemisphere, coronal section, is depicted)

Medial   Lateral

8.   A patient presents with significant weakness of the right leg from midcalf downward. He also has decreased sensory ability in the same area. Right Achilles reflex measure 3/4.
What is the source of the pathology? left anterior cerebral artery

9.   A patient presents with paralysis of the left arm, left upper body, and left face, with drooling as a result of inability to control the muscles around in left mouth. He also complains of decreased ability to "feel things" on the left face and arm.
What is the source of the pathology?   right middle cerebral artery

10.   A patient presents with hemiplegia of the entire right side of the body. Where is the pathology?   left internal capsule

11.   A patient presents with complaints of weakness of the hands and lower extremities. Muscle atrophy is evident in the feet and hands. Achilles deep tendon reflexes are increased. Brachioradialis flexes are decreased.
What is the likely diagnosis? ALS

12.   A patient presents right facial weakness and difficulty in moving eyes about voluntarily. On examination, she has a positive Romberg's sign. Babinski sign is present. Nystagmus is evident. She also complains of having had terrible difficulty in seeing things a couple weeks ago out of her left eye.
Where is the lesion? there is no one lesion – and all lesions are spread in space. Likely Dx = multiple sclerosis

13.   A patient suffered acute onset sharp back pain that started yesterday. The pain continues today, but the patient also states that he has "pins and needle" feelings on the bottom of his right foot. Achilles reflex is 1/4.
What is the likely neuro problem? radicular pathology due to impingement of S1 by L5 disc
What if he had no history of back pain, but rather a history of knee injury? What would you then consider as a possible neuro problem? impingement or damage to the tibial nerve (a branch of the sciatic nerve)

14.   A patient with a long history of various sexually transmitted diseases now presents with complaints of difficulty walking along with complaints of lancinating pain in his legs. He walks about by slamming his feet on the ground. On examination, he demonstrates a positive Romberg sign and decreased proprioception bilaterally in both legs.
What is the likely diagnosis? tabes dorsalis

KNOW YOUR DERMATOMES TO ALSO IDENTIFY RADICULAR PROBLEMS.

Radicular problems are motor or sensory problems that "radiate" from a damaged or injured nerve root. Common causes for radicular problems are herniated intervertebral discs, spinal cord tumors, tumors of spine, vertebral compression fractures, vertebral osteophytes, etc.

The major dermatomes include (e.g., sensory distribution):

C4	lateral shoulder
C5	lateral upper arm
C6	lateral forearm
C7	middle finger
C8	medial forearm
T1	medial upper arm
T10	band from T10 vertebral segment that wraps around body, dipping down to umbilicus
L1, 2, 3	anterior thigh
L4	knee and medial lower leg
L5	part of lateral lower leg below knee and above ankle + dorsum of foot
S1	plantar foot, lateral ankle, and strip up posteriolateral aspect of leg
S5	anus

Other helpful findings:

Signs of Disorders of the Cerebellum

Ataxia – inability to maintain balance; usually indicates cerebellar dysfunction

→ generally, people fall to the same side as the lesion

649

Dysmetria – overshooting the goal in reaching for an object
Scanning speech – awkward speech due to non-fluent control over muscles of speech
Dysdiadochokinesia – inability to perform rapid alternating movements like finger tapping
Decreased tendon reflexes – yes, decreased on the side affected can occur
Asthenia – muscle fatigue quickly
Intention tremor
Nystagmus

Signs of Disorders of the Basal Ganglia
Parkinsonism
Chorea
Athetosis
Hemiballismus – sudden, flailing movement of an arm

Section 109.0 Cardiovascular Anatomy

Section 109.1 Coronary Arteries

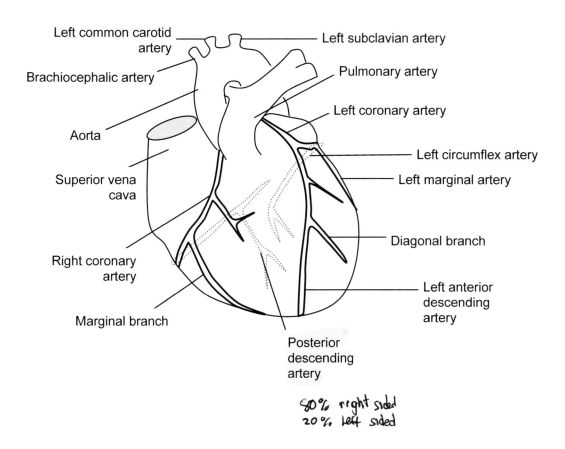

Left common carotid artery — Left subclavian artery
Brachiocephalic artery — Pulmonary artery
Aorta — Left coronary artery
Superior vena cava — Left circumflex artery
— Left marginal artery
Right coronary artery — Diagonal branch
Marginal branch — Left anterior descending artery
Posterior descending artery

80% right sided
20% left sided

- Right coronary artery (RCA) usually supplies the SA and AV nodes
- Marginal branch (acute marginal artery) supplies the right ventricle
- RCA, via the posterior descending artery (posterior interventricular artery; PDA), supplies the inferior left ventricle 80% of the time (20% of the time it is supplied by the left circumflex artery, and is known as left dominant supply)
- PDA supplies the posterior septum

Boards Boot Camp High-Yield Compendium

- Left anterior descending artery (LAD) supplies the anterior interventricular septum and the apex of the heart
- Left circumflex artery (LCX) supplies the left ventricle

➢ Coronary artery occlusion most commonly occurs in the LAD
➢ When the left main coronary artery is stenosed, it is colloquially known as the "widowmaker."

Heart Facts:

Blood supply = right and left coronary arteries, which are supplied by the aorta
- ✓ Left coronary supplies most of left atrium and ventricle, and anterior portion of the septum
- ✓ Right coronary supplies right atrium and ventricle, plus sinus and AV (atrioventricular) nodes
- ✓ Blood flow through coronary arteries is greatest during early diastole, and lowest during systole

Innervation = T1-6 (sympathetics) and vagus (parasympathetics)
- ✓ SA node usually receives its parasympathetic innervation from the right vagus
- ✓ AV node usually receives its parasympathetic innervation from the left vagus
- ✓ The atria are abundantly supplied by vagal innervation, whereas the ventricles are only sparsely innervated by the vagus
- ✓ The atria and ventricles are richly innervated by sympathetics

Origin = mesoderm

Section 109.1.1 Coronary Artery Lesions & Leads

EKG Leads	Cardiac Location	Coronary Vessel
V1-V3	Anteroseptal	RCA and/or LAD
V2-V4	Anterior	LAD
V4-V6	Anterolateral	LCA (widowmaker)
V5-V6	Lateral	LCX
I and aVL	High lateral	LCX
II,III, aVF	Inferior (Diaphragmatic)	RCA
V1-V3 with tall R waves + ST segment depression in V1-V3	Posterior	RCA and/or PDA
V1-V3 R wave reduction (MOST in V1), + V4-V6 S wave reduction, and V3R-V6R changes	Right ventricle	RCA with or without PDA

Key: RCA = right coronary artery; LAD = left anterior descending artery; LCA = left coronary artery; LCX = left circumflex artery; PDA = posterior descending artery

(Reprinted, with permission, from Dolinski, LA. *Boards Boot Camp Hi-Yield Compendium: Cardiology,* 1st ed., Pennsylvania, Pro-Medica, 2011: 48)

Section 109.2 Endocrine Gland Anatomy

Section 109.2.1   Adrenal Gland

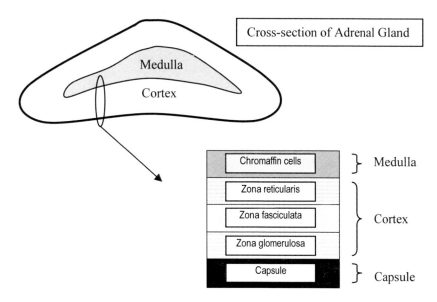

> Chromaffin cells are neuroendocrine cells; they are modified post-synaptic sympathetic neurons! They manage extreme sympathetic responses (by secreting epinephrine and norepinephrine)
> Zona reticularis manages sex (androgens)
> Zona fasciculata manages sugar (and WBCs, + lots more)
> Zona glomerulosa manages salt (Na, and water)
> The capsule is an adipose capsule

Adrenal Gland Facts:
Blood supply = superior, middle, and inferior suprarenal arteries
Innervation of cortex = T10,11 (sympathetics) and vagus (parasympathetics)
Innervation of medulla = celiac ganglion
Origin = mesoderm for cortex, neural crest for medulla

Section 109.2.2 Thyroid Gland

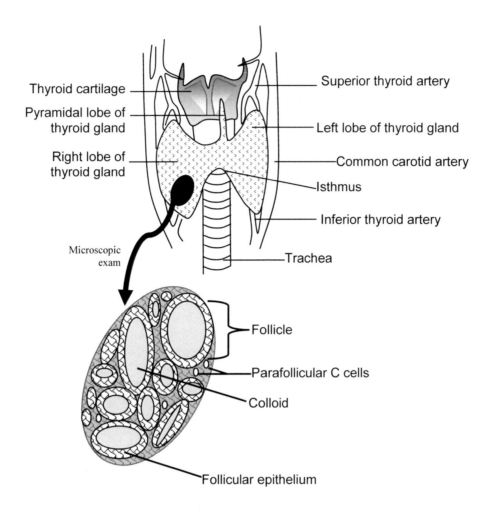

- Follicles absorb iodine ions from the blood to form, via the follicular epithelium, colloid; colloid is contained within the follicle
- Colloid is also known as thyroglobulin.
- Follicular epithelial cells are also known as follicular cells or thyrocytes.
- When stimulated by TSH (thyroid stimulating hormone), follicular epithelial cells re-absorb thyroglobulin to synthesize thyroxine (T4) and triiodothyronine (T3).

- The active form of T3 is made in the thyroid gland and also outside of the thyroid gland with the action of 5'-deiodinase.
- Parafollicular C cells produce calcitonin

  ➤ During thyroid surgery, risk of injury to the recurrent laryngeal nerves is prominent; at the inferior pole of the gland, the right recurrent laryngeal nerve is in close proximity to the inferior thyroid artery. Damage to the left is not as likely. Simple manipulation or injury of the right recurrent laryngeal nerve can result in temporary post-op laryngeal spasms or dysphonia (impaired voice production)
  ➤ Thyroidectomy also jeopardizes the parathyroid glands, 4 small glands that lie between the posterior thyroid and its sheath; they risk damage or accidental removal during the surgical process, resulting in primary hypoparathyroidism.

<u>Thyroid Gland Facts:</u>
Blood supply = superior and inferior thyroid arteries +/- thyroid ima artery
Innervation = T1-4 conducted through the superior, middle, and inferior cervical sympathetic ganglia (sympathetics) and vagus (parasympathetics)
Origin = 2nd branchial arch derived from endoderm for follicular cells, neural crest for parafollicular C cells

Section 109.2.3   Pituitary Gland

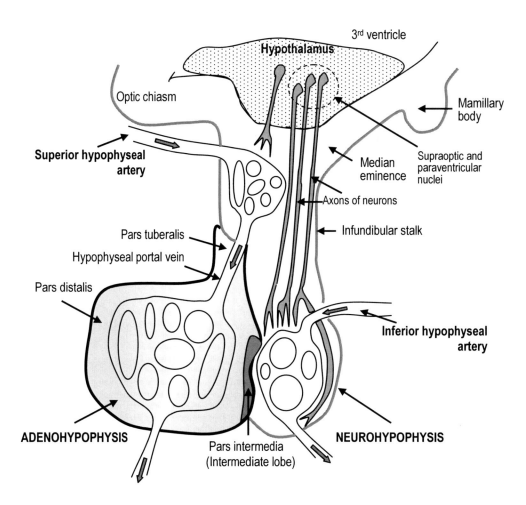

- The adenohypophysis is also known as the anterior pituitary gland or anterior lobe of the pituitary gland

- The adenohypophysis is comprised of 3 parts: pars distalis (the largest part; the "bulbous" part), pars tuberalis, and the pars intermedia; the adenohypophysis is a true gland

Boards Boot Camp High-Yield Compendium

- The neurohypophysis is also known as the posterior pituitary gland, the posterior lobe of the pituitary gland, or the pars nervosa; it is actually not glandular. It is a cluster of axons and nerve terminals from the hypothalamus.

- The pituitary gland sits in the sella turcica of the sphenoid bone of the skull

- The superior hypophyseal artery supplies the capillary bed in the median eminence. The capillaries provide increased surface area to serve nerve endings of axons extending from the hypothalamus; these nerve endings release a variety of releasing or inhibiting hormones, including TRH, CRH, etc. Then, these hormones are conducted from that capillary bed via the hypophyseal portal vein, down into the pars distalis of the anterior pituitary gland. This pituitary portal system ensures that the releasing and inhibitory hormones provided by the hypothalamus are not diluted in the blood stream. They are delivered, undiluted, throughout the anterior pituitary, allowing for maximal inhibition or stimulation by those hormones. The pituitary cells in the anterior pituitary then, in response to the hypothalamic hormones, synthesize, store, and eventually release (or are inhibited to synthesize and release) hormones into its own capillary bed, for eventual delivery to target organs systemically.

- Negative or positive feedback from target organs that ultimately controls the anterior pituitary is achieved by delivery of target organ hormones to the hypothalamus as well as, via the superior hypophyseal artery, to the anterior pituitary. Portal veins transport the hormones, in the latter case, throughout the anterior pituitary.

- Nerve cell bodies in the hypothalamus produce oxytocin and ADH (anti-diuretic hormone; vasopressin). These hormones are packaged into secretory granules, and passed down the long axons into the pars nervosa (posterior pituitary). The hormones are released by the terminal nerve endings into the pars nervosa, for storage and eventual release into its capillary bed.

- When the contents of granules destined for release in the pars nervosa are not immediately secreted, the granules can accumulate in groups as expansions or "lumps" along the axon; these expansions with accumulated numbers of granules within the axon are known as "Herring bodies."

Summary:
  ➢ Anterior pituitary makes, stores, and releases hormones; it does this under the influence of hypothalamic hormones
  ➢ Posterior pituitary only stores and releases hormones, the latter all being made and provided by the hypothalamus
  ➢ Anterior pituitary makes, stores and releases prolactin, ACTH, TSH, GH, FSH, and LH.
  ➢ Posterior pituitary stores and releases hypothalamic hormones, specifically oxytocin and ADH.

Notes:

The are several different cell types in the pituitary; they are categorized by how they stain for microscopic evaluation.

ACIDOPHILS: stain pink/red/orange
    Somatotropes – make growth hormone
    Lactotropes – make prolactin

BASOPHILS: stain blue/purple
    Corticotropes – makes POMC (pro-opiomelanocortin), and
        all of its by-products (including ACTH)
    Gonadotropes – make FSH and LH
    Thyrotropes – make TSH

Chromophobes are degranulated acidophils or basophils. They are colorless.

The pars distalis contains all types of acidophils, basophils, and chromophobes. The pars tuberalis contains some gonadotropes and/or thyrotropes. The pars intermedius contains some corticotropes.

The pars nervosa contains only axons and terminal nerve endings from the paraventricular and supraoptic nuclei of the hypothalamus.

Pituitary Gland Facts:
Blood supply = superior and inferior hypophyseal artery, which are branches of the internal carotid artery
Innervation = posterior pituitary is comprised of axons itself, plus glial cells – so it is nervous tissue; the cell bodies of these axons reside in the hypothalamus (supraoptic nuclei and paraventricular nuclei). Anterior pituitary is supplied by axons from the hypothalamus, but receives innervation via T1-4 (sympathetics).
Origin = neural ectoderm for posterior pituitary gland; oral ectoderm forms Rathke's pouch, from which the anterior pituitary gland (all three parts) is derived.

Boards Boot Camp High-Yield Compendium

Section 109.3 Retroperitoneal Anatomy

The retroperitoneum is the space that lies posterior to the peritoneal cavity, directly behind the peritoneum. The retroperitoneal structures include:

- o Aorta
- o Esophagus (lower 2/3)
- o Duodenum (excluding the first part)
- o Pancreas (excluding the tail of the pancreas)
- o Inferior vena cava
- o Adrenal glands
- o Kidneys
- o Ureters
- o Ascending and descending large intestine
- o Rectum (upper 2/3)

Section 109.4 Gastrointestinal System Anatomy

Section 109.4.1 Layers of Small Intestine Wall

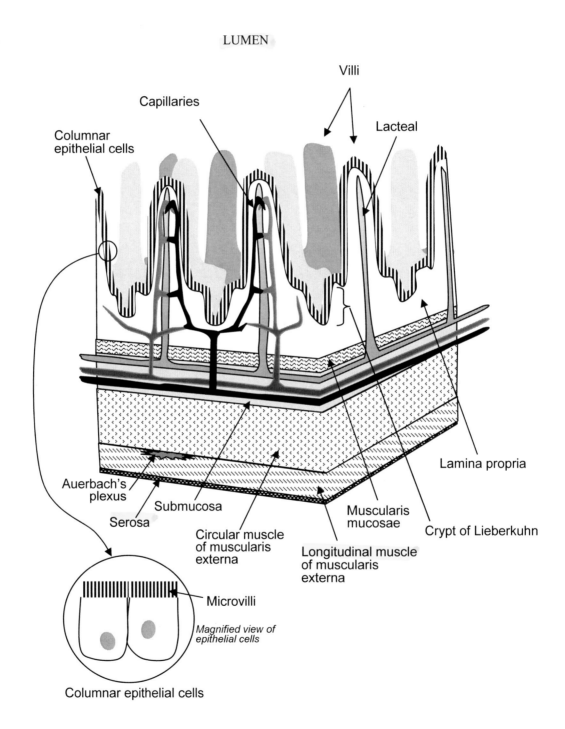

Boards Boot Camp High-Yield Compendium

- **Villi** serve to increase surface area for absorption as nutrients pass through the small bowel lumen. Surface area is further increased by microvilli.

- **Microvilli** are also known as the brush border.

- Microvilli are cellular extension protruding from the surface of the epithelial cells lining the villi.

- Microvilli are covered by plasma membrane and have, at their core, a dense bundle of actin filaments. The core of actin is linked to the overlying plasma membrane via myosin and calmodulin, and is anchored at its base to the cell's cytoskeleton proteins, mostly spectrin and myosin II. It is believed that the actin core may be capped on its apex (tip) with capZ proteins.

- Microvilli are covered, external to their overlying plasma membrane, with glycocalyx comprised of glycoproteins.

- The **columnar epithelial cells** providing the inner lining of the bowel are known as **enterocytes** or **absorptive cells**.

- The nutrients that are absorbed enter the enterocytes.

- In the small intestine lumen, **lipids**, in the form of monoglycerides and free fatty acids (by-products of pancreatic lipase-catalyzed triglyceride hydrolysis), cholesterol, and phospholipids, are dissolved in the center lipophilic portion of **bile acid micelles**. The micelles carry the lipids to the microvilli where the lipids easily diffuse into the enterocyte. These lipids eventually are packaged within the cell into chylomicrons. The chylomicrons then pass into the lymph of the **lacteals**, the smallest vessels of the lymphatic system. From there the lymph, complete with its **chylomicrons**, travels via the **lymphatics**, entering ever-larger lymphatic vessels, then the thoracic duct, from which it is finally emptied into the bloodstream at the subclavian vein.

- Bile acid micelles ensure that about 97% of fat is absorbed, while only about 40-50% is absorbed in the absence of such micelles.

- **Carbohydrates** (in the form of monosaccharides) and **proteins** (in the form of di- and tri-peptides, along with free amino acids) that are absorbed also enter the enterocytes (via Na co-transport, in most cases), and eventually enter the blood stream by way of the capillaries of the villi; from there, those nutrients are delivered by the **hepatic venous portal system**, being delivered eventually into the portal vein and finally into the liver. This allows for **first pass metabolism**. (Note that chylomicrons and other lipids can avoid first pass metabolism via bypassing the portal system and being, eventually, delivered to the systemic venous system).

- A few amino acids, as well as fructose, do not utilize the Na co-transport mechanism; they, instead, are transported into the enterocytes by special membrane transport proteins in a process known as **facilitated diffusion**.

- **Short- and medium-chain fatty acids**, such as what is found in butterfat (in butter), are able to diffuse into enterocytes and, as re-constituted short- and medium-chain triglycerides (SCTs and MCTs, respectively), diffuse directly from the enterocytes they have entered and into the capillary blood of the villi. This allows for delivery of certain fats to the liver via the portal system

> **Clinical Note:** Cow and goat milk is rich in SCTs. SCTs are also derived from the fermentation of dietary fiber in the colon. Short chain fatty acids (SCFAs, the components of SCTs), themselves, enhance healthy colonic flora and also provide a major source of energy for colonocytes (epithelial cells of the colon). Accordingly, studies have shown that specific SCFAs may reduce the risk for development of GI cancers and other GI disorders.
> Human milk, coconut oil, and palm kernel oil contain MCTs. MCTs are often used to supplement the diet of those with malabsorptive disorders, and are used in total parenteral nutrition (TPN). There is growing interest in the use of MCTs in controlling epilepsy and neurodegenerative disorders, such as Alzheimer's, and evidence that MCTs, unlike long-chain triglycerides (the typical fats we ingest), are linked to lower incidence of ischemic heart disease. MCTs as a fat source have also been shown to be effective in weight loss and decreasing serum triglyceride levels.

- The **lamina propria** is comprised of loose connective tissue, and contains glands with ducts that open into the intestine, allowing for secretion of mucus and serous secretions. There is also a rich population of lymphocytes, mostly **IgA-secreting plasma cells**, in the lamina propria.

- The lamina propria may also house **lymph nodules** that act as germinal centers where lymphocytes proliferate; these are particularly well-developed and evident as **Peyer's patches**, found in children and young adults in the ileum.

- The **muscularis mucosae** is a thin layer of smooth muscle. It agitates and "moves" the tissue, enhancing release of crypt of Lieberkuhn contents and increasing contact between brush border and lumen contents.

- The **crypts of Lieberkuhn** are also known as intestinal glands. They secrete a variety of enzymes, including sucrose, maltase, and enteropeptidase.

- The base of the intestinal glands contain stem cells which help to replenish lost cells of the villi and serve to create **goblet cells** (glandular columnar epithelial cells which secrete mucin which, when dissolved in water, forms **mucus**).

- The **mucosa** = epithelium + lamina propria + muscularis mucosae

- The **submucosa** lies deep to the mucosa, and contains lymphatics, blood vessels, and the **submucosal plexus** (also known as **Meissner's plexus**).

- Meissner's plexus is comprised of post-ganglionic nerve fibers of the parasympathetic nervous system, and serves the muscularis mucosae

667

- The muscularis externa is also known as the **muscularis propria** or the **muscular layer**.

- The muscularis externa is comprised of two separate layers of smooth muscle: the **circular layer and the longitudinal layer**.

- **Auerbach's plexus**, also known as the **myenteric plexus**, is located between the circular and longitudinal muscle of the muscularis externa. It is comprised of post-ganglionic parasympathetic fibers that work to coordinate contraction of the layers for **peristalsis**.

- The **serosa** consists of connective tissue with a surface of **mesothelium**, and has the same composition as mesentery.

- Mesothelium is simple squamous epithelium that forms the "outer surface" of the serosa of major body cavities (peritoneal, pericardial, and pleural).

- **Mesentery** is comprised of sheets of connective tissue which bind the loops of bowel together, and have the same composition as serosa (including a mesothelium on their exposed surfaces).

- The serosa comprises what is known as the **visceral peritoneum**, and continues over the abdominal wall as the **parietal peritoneum**.

Section 109.4.2 Layers of Large Intestine Wall

LUMEN

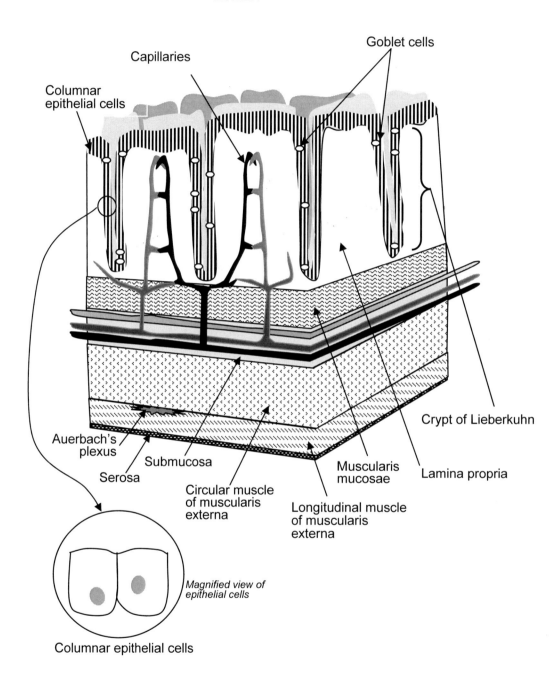

Capillaries

Goblet cells

Columnar epithelial cells

Auerbach's plexus

Serosa

Submucosa

Circular muscle of muscularis externa

Longitudinal muscle of muscularis externa

Muscularis mucosae

Lamina propria

Crypt of Lieberkuhn

Magnified view of epithelial cells

Columnar epithelial cells

- Notice that there are no villi.

- The cells on the luminal side of the mucosa are **simple columnar epithelium**, also termed **absorptive cells**. They do not have microvilli.

- Structurally, there are many similarities between the large intestine wall and small intestine wall, with the exception of lack of villi, lack of a brush border on the epithelial cells, abundance of goblet cells, depth of crypts, and absence of lacteals.

- There are abundant **goblet cells**; they carry out the same function as in the small intestine.

- The **crypts of Lieberkuhn** are very deep; they carry out a function similar to that in the small intestine.

- The **lamina propria** houses relatively large numbers of lymphocytes and other immune cells; in fact, it may also include scattered lymph nodules (germinal centers where lymphocytes proliferate), especially in the **appendix**.

Section 109.5 Skeletal Muscle System Anatomy

Section 109.5.1 Skeletal Muscle of the Tongue

Muscle	Innervation	Function
Genioglossus	**CN XII**	Sticks tongue out
Hypoglossus	**CN XII**	Lowers/pulls down tongue
Palatoglossus	CN X	Raises posterior tongue
Styloglossus	**CNXII**	Pulls sides of tongue up, pulls tongue inward

➤ CN XII = cranial nerve 12 = **hypoglossal nerve**

➤ **Hypoglossal nerve damage** allows contralateral genioglossus muscle (e.g., on undamaged side) to become the dominant muscle. Result = when patient is asked to stick their tongue out, it will deviate TOWARDS the side of damage. This is because the unaffected side will have a strong genioglossus, sticking the tongue out strongly, while the damaged side will not be able to push the tongue out as well, causing the tongue to deviate towards that damaged side.

➤ CN X = cranial nerve 10 = **vagus nerve**

➤ The **palatoglossus** is the ONLY muscle of the tongue not innervated by CN XII

> **Clinical Note:** The genioglossus, along with the geniohyoideus, help to maintain stability and patency of portions of the upper airway. Relaxation of these muscles during REM sleep is implicated in obstructive sleep apnea (OSA).

Section 109.5.2 Skeletal Muscle of the Jaw

Muscle	Innervation	Function
Lateral pterygoid (also known as external pterygoid)	**V3 of CN V**	**Opens mouth** + causes side-to-side movement of jaw + protrudes jaw
Digastric (has 2 bellies: anterior and posterior)	Anterior belly: **V3 of CN V** Posterior belly: CN VII	**Opens mouth**
Geniohyoid (also known as geniohyoideus)	CN XII	**Opens mouth** + aids in propelling food from mouth to pharynx
Masseter	V3 of CN V	**Closes mouth**
Medial pterygoid	V3 of CN V	**Closes mouth**
Temporalis (also known as the temporal)	**V3 of CN V**	**Closes mouth** + retracts jaw

◊ CN V = cranial nerve 5 = **trigeminal nerve**

◊ CN V has three branches: **V1** (ophthalmic nerve), **V2** (maxillary nerve), and **V3 (mandibular nerve)**

◊ **V3** is the only branch that has both sensory and motor functions (V1 and V2 have only sensory function)

◊ The motor function of V3 is innervation and control of the muscles of mastication (+ tensor tympani, tensor veli palatini, mylohyoid, and anterior belly of the digastric muscle).

◊ **The muscles of mastication** = masseter + medial pterygoid + lateral pterygoid + temporalis; the digastric is an accessory muscle of mastication

◊ Mastication means **to chew**

◊ The muscles of mastication originate embryologically from the **1ˢᵗ branchial arch** (as opposed to the muscles of facial expression, innervated by CN VII, which originate from the 2ⁿᵈ branchial arch).

Clinical Note: In tetanus, it is the muscles of mastication that develop severe, unrelenting painful spasms and tetany to cause "lockjaw" (trismus); these muscles are generally the first to suffer such tetany during the disease. Eventually spasms affect more muscles in a descending pattern. Tetany of the respiratory muscles eventually occurs, resulting in death.

Section 109.5.3 Skeletal Muscle of the Larynx

Muscle	Innervation	Function
Cricothyroid	**SUPERIOR** laryngeal nerve	Tenses the vocal cords
Lateral crico**arytenoid** (also known as the anterior cricoarytenoids)	**Recurrent laryngeal nerve**	Closes glottis
Posterior crico**arytenoid**	**Recurrent laryngeal nerve**	Opens glottis
Thyro**arytenoid**	**Recurrent laryngeal nerve**	Relaxes vocal cords

- The **cricothyroid muscle** aids with phonation; its contraction results in higher pitched phonation

- The superior laryngeal nerve is a branch of the **vagus**

673

- The **superior laryngeal nerve** is responsible for **motor control of the cricothyroid**, and for **sensory ABOVE the glottis.**

- **Superior laryngeal nerve palsy**, which can result from injury such as through thyroidectomy, causes a hoarse, lower voice that easily tires.   on Ⓡ

- **Thyroarytenoid muscle** contraction relaxes the vocal cords, decreasing the pitch of the voice

- The **recurrent laryngeal nerve** is a branch of the vagus

- The recurrent laryngeal nerve provides **sensory innervation to the larynx BELOW the glottis**, and supplies all laryngeal muscles except the cricothyroid.

- The recurrent laryngeal nerve is "recurrent" because it branches off from the vagus, descends into the chest, and ascends again ("recurs"), providing innervation to the larynx.

- The **left recurrent laryngeal nerve** branches off from the vagus, and then **loops under the aortic arch** before ascending.

- The **right recurrent laryngeal nerve** branches off from the vagus, and then **loops under the right subclavian artery** before ascending.

- Neck injury, thyroidectomy, chest tumors, or even aneurysms (such as of the aortic arch) can impair recurrent laryngeal nerve function.

> **Clinical Note:** Unilateral dysfunction of the recurrent laryngeal nerve, such as can occur with aortic arch aneurysms, chest tumors, and injury via thyroidectomy or carotid endarterectomy typically cause voice changes, most notably hoarseness. Bilateral damage, such as through trauma, will impair patency of the larynx, yielding aphonia (the inability to produce any sounds of voice) and, in the worst cases, asphyxia.

Section 109.5.4 Skeletal Muscle of the Neck:
KEY MUSCLES

Muscle	Classification	Innervation	Function
Sternocleidomastoid	Cervical muscle	CN XI (for motor) *Cervical plexus (from C2-3) provides sensory*	*Unilateral contraction:* **Ipsilateral sidebending of neck** with contralateral head rotation *Bilateral contraction:* **Neck flexion, + forced inspiration**
Anterior scalene muscles	Lateral vertebral muscles	C5, C6, C7, C8	Elevates 1st rib *Unilateral contraction:* **Ipsilateral sidebending of neck** with contralateral head rotation *Bilateral contraction:* **Neck flexion, + forced inspiration**

Boards Boot Camp High-Yield Compendium

Posterior scalene muscles	Lateral vertebral muscles	C5, C6, C7, C8	Elevates 2nd rib *Unilateral contraction:* **Ipsilateral sidebending of neck** *Bilateral contraction:* **Neck flexion, + forced inspiration**
Middle scalene muscles	Lateral vertebral muscles	C3, C4	Elevates 1st rib *Unilateral contraction:* **Ipsilateral sidebending of neck** *Bilateral contraction:* **Neck flexion, + forced inspiration**

Section 109.5.5 Skeletal Muscle of the Shoulder & Scapula: KEY MUSCLES

Muscle	Innervation	Function
Supraspinatus	Suprascapular nerve (C4, 5)	**Abduction of arm** (is the main agonist during the 1st 10-15 degree, and is THE initiator of abduction)
Serratus anterior	Long thoracic nerve (C5, 6, 7)	**Aids arm abduction** (by rotating scapula) **+** protracts (brings forward) scapula
Deltoid	Axillary nerve (C5, 6)	**Abduction of arm** (is the main agonist beyond 30 degrees) **+** <u>Arm flexion</u> **+** Arm extension
Infraspinatus	Suprascapular nerve (C5, 6)	**External rotation of arm** (outward rotation, lateral rotation)
Teres minor	Axillary nerve (C5, 6)	**External rotation of arm** (outward rotation, lateral rotation)
Subscapularis	Subscapular nerves (C5, 6)	**Internal rotation of arm** (inward rotation, medial rotation)
Pectoralis major	Pectoral nerves (C5, 6, 7, 8, and T1)	**Internal rotation of arm** + Adduction of arm + <u>Arm flexion</u> (clavicular head of muscle) **+** Arm Extension (sternocostal head of muscle)
Teres major	Lower subscapular nerve (C6, 7)	**Internal rotation of arm**

Levator scapulae	Cervical nerve (C3, 4) and Dorsal scapular nerve (C5)	**Rotates scapula down for good posture +** Elevates scapula
Rhomboid major	Dorsal scapular nerve (C4, 5)	**Rotates scapula down for good posture +** Retracts (brings back, posteriorly) scapula
Rhomboid minor	Dorsal scapular nerve (C4, 5)	**Rotates scapula down for good posture +** Retracts (brings back, posteriorly) scapula
Trapezius	CN XI (motor) + C2, C3 and C4 (motor and sensory)	Rotates, elevates, retracts, and depresses scapula + aids arm abduction
Pectoralis minor	Medial pectoral nerve (C8, T1)	Stabilizes the scapula by moving it inferiorly and anteriorly

- o **The rotator cuff** is comprised of a group of muscles, and their tendons; specifically, it is comprised of the supraspinatus, infraspinatus, teres minor, and the subscapularis. Although they work to move the arm in various ways, they are grouped together as "rotator cuff" muscles because they act to **stabilize the glenohumeral joint.**

- o The main muscles of **upper body posture maintenance** are the rhomboids, the levator scapulae, and the trapezius.

o **The deltoid and the supraspinatus are considered to work somewhat synergistically in arm abduction;** the supraspinatus initiates the abduction, and is the primary abductor up to about 15 degrees. The deltoid assists, having a gradually greater role in abduction with increasing arc, becoming the primary (but not only) abductor beyond 30 degrees. The supraspinatus contributes up to 90 degrees, but less and less as the degree of abduction is increased.

o **Rotator cuff tears** are any tear of the structures of the rotator cuff; the most common tear is a supraspinatus tendon tear.

o **Rotator cuff tears are usually of acute onset, following trauma.**

o **Supraspinatus tendonitis** is not a rotator cuff tear; it is **inflammation of the tendon** to the supraspinatus, and is most common to persons who do a lot of overhead work or movement (e.g., baseball pitchers, swimmers, tennis players)

o Supraspinatus tendonitis will produce a **painful arc** of motion secondary to **impingement of the highly inflamed tendon under, most commonly, the acromion and a rigid coracoacromial arch.** That is why the painful arc becomes most pronounced beyond 60 degrees of abduction – that is the position beyond which the tendon becomes gradually more impinged under those structures, thus producing pain.

679

o **Drop arm test** is helpful for supraspinatus pathology. Extreme pain during the drop arm test, or refusal to do it due to pain, is most indicative of supraspinatus tendonitis. A drop arm test wherein the arm just drops to the side is more indicative of a torn supraspinatus tendon (torn rotator cuff).

Section 109.5.6 Skeletal Muscle of the Elbow:
KEY MUSCLES

Muscle	Innervation	Function
Supinator	Radial nerve, via Posterior interosseus nerve (C5, 6)	Forearm supination
Biceps brachii	Musculocutaneous nerve (C5, 6)	**Forearm flexion +** Forearm supination
Brachialis	Musculocutaneous nerve (C5, 6)	**Forearm flexion**
Brachioradialis	Radial nerve (C5, 6)	**Forearm flexion**
Pronator teres	Median nerve (C6, 7)	**Forearm flexion +** *Forearm pronation*
Pronator quadratus	Median nerve (C7-8, T1)	*Forearm pronation*
Triceps brachii	Radial nerve (C6-C8, T1)	Forearm extension (and long head aids in adduction and extension of the arm at the shoulder)

- The **primary flexor** of the forearm is the brachialis.

- The **primary extensor** of the forearm is the triceps.

- The **primary supinators** of the forearm are the biceps and the supinator.

- The **primary pronators** are the pronator teres and the pronator quadratus.

Why are different nerve roots listed with the same nerve for innervation of particular muscles?

Because one nerve is formed from contribution of typically multiple nerve roots; but certain nerve roots contribute more or less to that nerve's innervation of a particular muscle. For instance, the radial nerve is derived from C5-T1 nerve roots. However, the nerve root contributions <u>in</u> the radial nerve that most influence control over the brachioradialis are C5-C6, while those with most influence over the triceps are C6-C8 and T1, even though both muscles are innervated by the same nerve, specifically the radial nerve. Also, while many nerve root contributions within one nerve can influence control over a muscle, their individual influence on that muscle may not be even. For instance, while the radial nerve innervates the triceps, it is the fibers in that nerve that are derived from nerve roots C6-8 and T1 that do so. However, do all of those fibers have equal influence or control over the muscle? No. The fibers derived from C7 have the greatest influence, which is why triceps reflex testing is used to test primarily C7.

Boards Boot Camp High-Yield Compendium

Section 109.5.7 Skeletal Muscle of the Fingers and Wrist:
KEY FLEXOR MUSCLES

Muscle	Innervation	Function
Flexor carpi radialis	Median nerve (C6, C7)	**Flexes wrist +** Abducts wrist
Palmaris longus	Median nerve (C6, C7)	**Flexes wrist**
Flexor digitorum superficialis	Median nerve (C7, C8, T1))	**Flexes wrist +** *Flexes PIP joints*
Flexor digitorum profundus	Median nerve, via anterior interosseous branch (C7-8, T1) and Ulnar nerve (C7-C8, T1)	**Flexes wrist +** *Flexes PIP joints +* Flexes MCP and DIP joints
Flexor carpi ulnaris	Ulnar nerve (C8, T1)	**Flexes wrist +** Adducts wrist
Flexor **pollicis** longus	Median nerve, via anterior interosseous branch (C6-8, T1)	Flexes thumb at interphalangeal joint

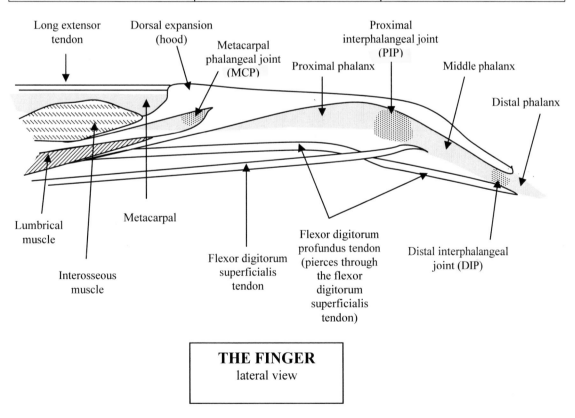

THE FINGER
lateral view

Section 109.5.8 Skeletal Muscle of the Hip:
KEY MUSCLES

Hamstring

Muscle	Innervation	Function
Semimembranosus	Tibial nerve (L4-5, S1-2)	**Extends thigh at hip +** Adducts thigh + *Medially rotates thigh +* Medially rotates leg at knee + Flexion of leg at knee
Semitendinosus	Tibial nerve (L4-5, S1-2)	**Extends thigh at hip +** Adducts thigh + *Medially rotates thigh +* Medially rotates leg at knee
Biceps femoris	Tibial nerve (L5, S1-3) and Common peroneal nerve (L5, S1-2)	**Extends thigh at hip +** Abducts thigh + *Laterally rotates thigh +* Flexion of leg at knee
Gluteus maximus	Inferior gluteal nerve (S1 mostly, + L4-5, S2)	**Extends thigh at hip +** Abducts thigh
Gluteus medius	Superior gluteal nerve (L5 mostly, + L4, S1)	Abducts thigh + *Medially rotates thigh*
Gluteus minimis	Superior gluteal nerve (L4-5, S1)	Abducts thigh + *Medially rotates thigh +* **Aids hip flexion +** Lateral hip stabilizer
Adductor magnus	Obturator and Sciatic nerves (L2, 3, 4, 5, S1)	Adducts thigh + **Aids Extension of thigh at hip +** Aids Flexion of thigh at hip + *Laterally rotates thigh*
Adductor minimus	Obturator nerve	Adducts thigh + *Laterally rotates thigh*

683

Iliospoas	Branches of femoral plexus (L1) and Femoral nerve (L2, 3)	**Flexes thigh at hip**
Quadriceps	Femoral nerve (L2, 3, 4)	**Flexes thigh at hip +** Extension of leg at knee

❖ The **quadriceps** are also known as the quadriceps femoris, or simply, the quads.

❖ The quads is a large muscle group that includes 4 muscles within it: **rectus femoris** (middle of anterior thigh), **vastus lateralis** (lateral anterior thigh), **vastus medialis** (medial anterior thigh), and **vastus intermedius** (between vastus medialis and lateralis, behind the rectus femoris).

❖ Besides playing important roles in movement at the hip and knee, the quads are also critical to **stabilization of the patella.**

❖ The **femoral nerve** supplies a number of muscles, including the iliopsoas and the quadriceps.

❖ The femoral nerve is the **largest nerve branch of the lumbar plexus**, and is comprised of L2, L3, and L4.

❖ The **iliopsoas** is comprised of two muscles: the psoas major and the iliacus.

❖ The **iliopsoas origin is T12-L5**. Thus, contraction or spasm, such as seen with iliopsoas flexion contracture, can cause vertebral segment flexion, with ipsilateral sidebending and rotation.

❖ **Iliopsoas contracture** is also known as **psoas syndrome**.

❖ It occurs most frequently in those who perform **prolonged or repeated hip flexion movements**; it can be seen in gardeners, gymnasts, and dancers.

❖ Iliopsoas contracture causes pain in the hip and thigh which is **exacerbated when the leg at the hip is straightened.**

❖ The **sciatic nerve** is the largest nerve in the body.

❖ The sciatic nerve supplies sensory to the skin of the posterior thigh and gluteal regions, as well as the entire lower leg (except for the medial leg)

❖ The sciatic nerve is derived from the **lumbar and sacral plexuses,** specifically L4-S3
    Tx-L4
    L5-S4

❖ The gluteal region is a common site for **intramuscular (IM) injections** – but there is risk of sciatic nerve injury; to prevent that, injections MUST be made in the upper lateral quadrant of the region

❖ The **gluteus maximus** is the largest of the three gluteal muscles. It makes up, along with fat, the bulk of the shape of the buttocks.

❖ The **common peroneal nerve** is also known as the **common fibular nerve**, the external popliteal nerve, or just the peroneal nerve.

Boards Boot Camp High-Yield Compendium

❖ A **posterior fibular head** can compress the peroneal nerve, leading to foot drop and weakened dorsiflexion of the foot, along with sensory disturbance on the dorsal foot.

❖ The **hamstrings** are comprised of the **biceps femoris**, the **semimembranosus**, and the **semitendinosus**.

Clinical Note:

<u>Psoas abscess</u> is a pus-filled abscess in the psoas muscle of the iliopsoas. Given the extreme proximal location of the psoas next to the vertebral bodies, abdominal aorta, sigmoid colon, appendix, and hip joint, infections in any of those locations can spread contiguously to the muscle, leading to an abscess. It causes abdominal, groin, or low back pain, plus often fever.

<u>Sciatica</u> typically causes radiating pain in the posterior lateral leg and posterior lateral buttocks region; it produces a positive Straight Leg Raising test and Bragard's test. It has many causes, including disc herniation, spinal stenosis, pregnancy, and piriformis syndrome.

<u>Neurolathyrism</u> is a neurodegenerative disease common to areas that are suffering famine. It is caused by eating grass pea or blue sweet pea seeds, which grow abundantly even during times of drought and can often be the only source of nutrients for extended periods of time. The seed contains a neurotoxin that results in severe atrophy of all gluteal muscles. It has been seen throughout history, and continues to be a problem in parts of Africa and the Middle East.

<u>Peroneal neuropathy</u> is any pathology of the peroneal nerve, and can be caused by a posterior fibular head, immobilization, and even habitual leg crossing; it leads to problems with foot dorsiflexion and sensation on the dorsal foot.

What about the Terrible Triad?

➢ There are many different Terrible Triads, for different joints in the body

➢ There are two types of Terrible Triads for the knee:
O'Donahue's Triad
Shelbourne's Triad

➤ Contrary to medically misleading information by some other boards prep sources, Shelbourne's has NOT replaced O'Donahue's; both exist, just in different populations and in different numbers

➤ O'Donahue's triad = rupture of the MCL and ACL, with medial meniscus tear

➤ Shelbourne's triad = rupture of the MCL and ACL, with lateral meniscus tear

➤ Shelbourne's triad was described after a small, local study of only 60 knees. It is, therefore, considered a non-classical Terrible Triad.

➤ O'Donahue's, considered the standard in orthopedic texts as well as medical coding, is the classical Terrible Triad.

➤ So, what is the answer if you get this on boards? Remember, the O'Donahue triad is the classic, and being found in many more knees. So, if nothing else is provided, it is more likely,

➤ But...age plays a role. Shelbourne's triad is most common to pre-adolescents and adolescents, while O'Donahue's is much more common in adults.

Section 109.5.9 Skeletal Muscle of the Foot & Ankle: KEY MUSCLES

Muscle	Innervation	Function
Gastrocnemius	Tibial nerve (S1 mostly, with some L5)	**Plantar flexion +** Flexes knee
Soleus	Tibial nerve (L4-5, S1-2)	**Plantar flexion**
Tibialis posterior	Tibial nerve (L5, S1)	**Plantar flexion +** *Foot inversion*
Flexor digitorum longus	Tibial nerve (L5, S1)	**Plantar flexion +** *Foot inversion +* Plantar flexes DIPs, PIPs, & MTPs of 2nd-5th toes
Peroneus longus and brevis	Common peroneal nerve (S1 mostly, with some L4-5)	**Plantar flexion +** *Foot eversion*
Flexor **hallucis** longus	Tibial nerve (S1 mostly, with some L5 and S2)	Flexes great toe + **Assists plantar flexion**
Flexor digitorum brevis	Medial plantar nerve (L4, L5, S1)	Plantar flexes PIP joints of toes 2-5
Peroneus tertius	**Deep peroneal nerve** (L4-5, S1)	**Dorsiflexion +** *Foot eversion*
Tibialis anterior	**Deep peroneal nerve** (L4 mostly, with some L5, S1)	**Dorsiflexion +** *Foot inversion*
Extensor **hallucis** longus	**Deep peroneal nerve** (L5 mostly, with some L4, S1)	**Dorsiflexion +** *Foot inversion +* Dorsiflexes DIP joint of great toe
Extensor digitorum longus	**Deep peroneal nerve** (L5 mostly, with some L4, S1)	**Dorsiflexion +** *Foot eversion +* Dorsiflexes PIP joints of toes 2-5

✓ The gastrocnemius, in combination with the soleus, is the **calf muscle.**

✓ The gastrocnemius is particularly prone to spasms, colloquially sometime referred to as "**charley horses.**"

✓ The soleus plays an especially vital role in the **skeletal muscle pump,** the pump responsible for increasing venous return to the heart via muscle contraction.

✓ Besides the functions the tibialis posterior plays when contracted, its tonicity also strongly supports the **medial arch of the foot.**

✓ Damage to the tibialis posterior can result in **pes planus (flat foot),** with unopposed eversion.

✓ The tonicity of the peroneus longus helps to stabilize the **transverse arch of the foot.**

✓ The **deep peroneal nerve** is also known as the **deep fibular nerve.**

✓ The deep peroneal nerve is a branch of the **common peroneal nerve.**

✓ **Injury to the deep peroneal nerve** results in **foot drop** (loss of dorsiflexion).

✓ **Injury to the common peroneal nerve** results in foot drop PLUS sensory disturbance on the dorsal foot and lateral leg.

689

✓ **Injury to the tibial nerve** results in loss of plantar flexion of the foot and toes.

Section 109.6 <u>Must-Know Clinical Anatomy Facts</u>

1.   AV shunts (arteriovenous malformations) are often considered pathologic; however, they are present in great numbers normally throughout the skin of the nose, lips, fingers, and ears, where they conserve body heat.

2.   AV shunts (arteriovenous malformations) are areas in which there are no capillaries between the arterioles and venules, allowing for direct connection between those arterioles and venules.

3.   Sinusoids are wider and more irregular than capillaries, and take the place of capillaries in the liver, spleen, red bone marrow, adenohypophysis (anterior pituitary), suprarenal cortex, and parathyroid glands; their walls consist largely of phagocytic cells.

4.   A fracture at the distal end of the radius is a Colles' fracture.

5.   The rotator (musculotendinous) cuff is comprised of the subscapularis, supraspinatus, infraspinatus, and teres minor muscles.

6.   The mammary gland is a modified sweat gland that is located in the superficial fascia.

7.   The breast has suspensory ligaments (Cooper's ligaments) that support the breast and run from the dermis to the deep layer of the superficial fascia through the breast.

8.   As breast cancer encroaches on and /or attaches to Cooper's ligaments, these ligaments are shortened; this causes dimpling of the overlying skin.

9.   As breast cancer attaches to and shortens the lactiferous ducts, it can cause a retracted or inverted nipple.

10.   A radical mastectomy is the removal of the breast, pectoralis major and minor muscles, axillary lymph nodes and fascia, and part of the thoracic wall.

11.   A modified radical mastectomy is the removal of the breast and axillary lymph nodes.

12.   Pectoralis minor muscle runs from the 2nd to the 5th ribs and is innervated mainly by the medial pectoral nerve (and, to a lesser extent, by the lateral pectoral nerve).

13.   The pectoralis major muscle runs from the medial half of the clavicle, the manubrium and body of the sternum, and the upper 6 costal cartilages, and is innervated by the lateral and medial pectoral nerves.

14.   Structures inside the carpal tunnel include the median nerve and the tendons of the flexor pollicis longus, flexor digitorum profundus, and flexor digitorum superficialis muscles.

15.   The anatomical snuff box is bounded by the tendon of the extensor pollicis longus muscle and the tendons of the extensor pollicis brevis and abductor pollicis longus muscles.

16.   The dorsal (extensor) expansion of the digits is an expansion of the extensor tendon that is over the dorsal MCP; it is termed the "extensor hood." It provides the insertion of the interossei and lumbricals.

17.   Dorsal interossei abduct the fingers while the palmar interossei adduct the fingers. The lumbricals flex the MCP joints and extend the PIP and DIP joints.

18.   The brachial plexus arises from C5-T1 nerve roots. It passes between the anterior and middle scalene muscles. It is enclosed with the axillary artery and vein in the axillary sheath.

19.   Dorsal scapular nerve (C5)   Long thoracic nerve (C5-C7)
        Suprascapular nerve (C5-C6)   Nerve to subclavius (C5)
        Lateral pectoral n. (C5-C7)   Musculocutaneous n. (C5-C7)
        Medial pectoral nerve (C8-T1)   Medial brachial cutaneous n. (C8-T1)
        Medial antebrachial cutaneous n. (C8-T1) Ulnar n. (C7-T1)
        Upper subscapular n. (C5-C6)   Thoracodorsal n. (C7-C8)
        Lower subscapular n. (C5-C6)   Axillary nerve (C5-C6)
        Radial n. (C5-T1)   Musculocutaneous n. (C5-C7)
        Median n. (C5-T1)

20.   The cell bodies of the general somatic and general visceral afferents are in the dorsal root ganglia.

21.   The cell bodies of the general somatic efferents are in the anterior horn of the spinal cord.

22.   The cell bodies of the sympathetic postganglionic general visceral efferents are in the sympathetic chain ganglia.

23.   The suprascapular artery is a branch of the thyrocervical trunk, and anastomoses with the deep branch of the transverse cervical artery (dorsal scapular artery) and the circumflex scapular artery around the scapula (thereby providing a collateral circulation).

24. The axillary artery extends form the outer border of the first rib to the inferior border of the teres major muscle, where it becomes the brachial artery.

25. Fracture of the clavicle results in an upward displacement of the proximal fragment because of the pull of the sternocleidomastoid muscle. The downward displacement of the distal fragment is caused by the deltoid muscle and by gravity.

26. Fracture of the clavicle may result in lower trunk brachial plexus injury as well as fatal hemorrhages or thromboses of the subclavian vein.

27. A Colles'-like fracture that has the radial distal fragment displaced anteriorly (instead of posteriorly as in Colles') is known as a Reverse Colles' Fracture or as a Smith's fracture.

28. An inferior dislocation of the humerus is not uncommon because there is little support of the shoulder joint inferiorly; this dislocation may damage the axillary nerve and the posterior humeral circumflex artery.

29. Referred pain to the shoulder often indicates the involvement of the phrenic nerve or diaphragm; this is because the supraclavicular nerve (C3-C4) (supplies sensory fibers to the shoulder) has the same origin as the phrenic nerve (C3-C5) (supplies the diaphragm).

30. Carpal tunnel syndrome is caused by compression of the median nerve.

31. Fracture of the middle shaft of the humerus may result in injury to the radial nerve, leading to wrist drop.

32. Fracture of the medial epicondyle may result in injury to the ulnar nerve resulting in claw hand.

33. A supracondylar injury to the humerus may result in median nerve injury, with resultant ape hand.

34. The anterior cruciate ligament is in the knee joint capsule but external to the synovial cavity of the knee joint.

35. The anterior cruciate ligament prevents backward slipping of the femur on the tibia, and therefore limits excessive anterior mobility of the tibia on the femur when the knee is extended.

36. The posterior cruciate ligament is in the knee joint capsule but external to the synovial cavity.

37. The posterior cruciate ligament limits hyperflexion of the knee and prevents forward movement of the femur on the tibia.

38.   The medial (tibial) collateral ligament is firmly attached to the medial meniscus; therefore, damage to this ligament also invariably causes damage to the medial meniscus. This ligament also attaches to the medial aspects of the articular capsule and the tibial condyle.

39.   The lateral (fibular) collateral ligament is attached to the lateral femoral epicondyle and the head of the fibula.

40.   Obturator nerve – arises from the lumbar plexus from L3-L4
        Lumbar Plexus (T12-L4)
        Femoral nerve – arises from the lumbar plexus from L2-L4
        Sacral plexus (L4-S3)
        The superior and inferior gluteal nerves arise from the sacral plexus from
                L4-S1 and L5-S2, respectively.
        The sciatic nerve arises from the sacral plexus from L4-S3

41.   The largest nerve in the body is the sciatic nerve.

42.   The two parts of the sciatic nerve are the tibial and common peroneal (fibular) components.

43.   The obturator artery arises from the internal iliac artery.

44.   The femoral artery is the continuation of the external iliac artery distal to the inguinal ligament.

45.   The profunda femoris (deep femoral) artery arises from the femoral artery within the femoral triangle.

46.   The patellar reflex = knee-jerk reflex; occurs when patellar ligament is tapped, causing a sudden contraction of the quadriceps femoris; it tests L4.

47.   The ankle-jerk reflex is induced when the tendon calcaneus is tapped, resulting in contraction of the triceps surae (medial and lateral heads of the gastrocnemius and the soleus muscles); it tests S1.

48.   A femoral hernia is a sac formed by the parietal peritoneum that passes through the femoral ring and canal (i.e. lateral to the pubic tubercle and deep to the inguinal ligament); it is more common in women than men.

49.   Gluteal gait = Waddling Gait; it is characterized by falling of the pelvis to the unaffected side with each step. It is due to paralysis of the gluteus medius muscle. (This muscle usually functions to stabilize the pelvis when the opposite foot is off the ground.)

50.   Congenital dislocation of the hip joint results from abnormal development of the upper lip of the acetabulum; as such, the femoral head leaves the acetabulum and moves onto the gluteal surface of the ilium. The affected limb is shortened, adducted, and medially rotated.

51. Bleeding from the ear is a common finding in basilar skull fractures; Battle's sign is discoloration of the skin along the course of the posterior auricular artery (in the area of the mastoid), and is indicative of a basilar skull fracture.

52. The most common cause of death from a skull fracture is laceration of the brain.

53. Separation of the cranial bones at the fontanelles at birth allows the skull to adapt (or "mould") during passage through the birth canal.

54. The scalp has five layers: skin, subQ tissue, musculoaponeurotic tissue (galea aponeurotica and the frontalis and occipitalis muscles), subaponeurotic layer, and the pericranium (periosteum of the bones); this provides the acronym S C A L P.

55. The scalp pericranium (periosteum) is poorly connected to the bone by connective tissue known as Sharpey's fibers.

56. The galea aponeurotica unites the frontal and occipital muscles of the cranial vault.

57. Because the subaponeurotic layer is very loose, large amounts of blood can form huge hematomas after blows to the head.

58. Because of the looseness of the subaponeurotic layer, infections entering this layer spread easily and widely, eventually traveling by way of emissary veins (which pass through bones directly to the dura) and via diploic veins (which are located between the skull's bony tables).

59. Sebaceous cysts are wens, and represent obstruction of sebaceous gland ducts; they are commonly found on the scalp.

60. Infections on the face above the mouth can be carried into the cavernous sinus by way of the facial, angular, and superior ophthalmic veins.

61. Enlarged supraclavicular nodes on the left side are frequently associated associated with stomach and/colon cancer.

62. Inflammation of the walls of the emissary veins (i.e., secondary to infection) may lead to thrombophlebitis of the dural venous sinuses.

63. Damage to the facial nerve or its branches produces various degrees of weakness and/or paralysis of facial muscles, and is referred to as "Bell's palsy."

64. Paralysis of the entire side of the face indicates that the facial nerve itself has been damaged somewhere along its course. Forehead movement is maintained if the damage is in the cerebral cortex or the descending corticobulbar fibers rather than in the facial nucleus or the peripheral itself.

65. The masseter, temporalis, and medial pterygoid muscles serve to close the jaw.

66.   The lateral pterygoid, suprahyoid, and infrahyoid muscles serve to open the mouth.

67.   The posterior fibers of the temporalis muscle are the chief retractors of the jaw.

68.   When the lateral pterygoids are contracted unilaterally alternatively, they will move the jaw from side to side. If contracted bilaterally, they serve to open the mouth.

69.   Loss of taste on the anterior 2/3 of the tongue indicates chorda tympani nerve involvement.

70.   Damage to the nerve to the stapedius muscle may cause hyperacusis (exaggerated sense of noises).

71.   Trigeminal neuralgia (tic douloureux) causes excruciating pain, especially along the maxillary and mandibular divisions of the trigeminal nerve. It is sometimes treated with alcohol injections into the trigeminal ganglion or at the nerve root where it leaves the skull. More commonly, medications such as TCAs are used.

72.   Herpes zoster infections can involve each division of the 5th cranial nerve.

73.   The temporomandibular joint has an articular disk which divides the joint cavity into upper and lower parts.

74.   The carotid sheath surrounds the internal and common carotid arteries, the internal jugular vein, and the vagus nerve, and adheres to the thyroid sheath.

75.   The retropharyngeal space lies between the buccopharyngeal and prevertebral fascia. At its cephalad end, it ends at the skull. At its caudad end, it continues into the mediastinum. Laterally, it ends at the carotid sheath.

76.   A retropharyngeal abscess is an abscess that develops in the retropharyngeal space; it can cause dysphagia, dysarthria, and mediastinitis.

77.   When venous pressure increases (i.e., as in heart failure), the external jugular vein becomes prominent and is easily seen in the neck; it is termed jugular venous distention.

78.   The carotid sinus is a slightly dilated area in the proximal internal carotid artery; it is an arterial blood pressure-regulating area, and is innervated by CN IX mainly with supplemental innervation provided by CN X and sympathetics.

79. The carotid body is a body small, ovoid tissue at the bifurcation of the common carotid artery. It is a chemoreceptor that is sensitive to increased carbon dioxide or decreased oxygen. It is innervated by the carotid sinus nerve of CN IX, X, and sympathetics.

80. Subclavian steal syndrome is due to a narrowing of the left subclavian artery near its origin. To compensate for the decreased blood flow to the arm, blood flows from the right to the left vertebral artery and then into the left subclavian artery. This leads to less blood flow to the brain, resulting in giddiness, syncope, and left arm ischemia.

81. The brachiocephalic trunk is on the right of the thorax.

82. The brachiocephalic trunk bifurcates to create the common carotid artery and the right subclavian artery.

83. The first branch of the subclavian artery is the vertebral artery.

84. The second branch off of the subclavian artery is the thyrocervical trunk.

85. The third branch off of the subclavian artery is the costocervical trunk.

86. The 4th branch off of the subclavian artery is the descending (dorsal) scapular artery.

87. The subclavian artery passes between the anterior and middle scalene muscles, along with the brachial plexus.

88. The subclavian vein passes anteriorly to the anterior scalene muscle.

89. After passing the anterior scalene muscle, both the subclavian artery and vein pass underneath the clavicle, along with the brachial plexus.

90. Any pathologic enlargement of the thyroid gland is known as a goiter.

91. A thyroglossal duct may persist and remain patent between the foramen cecum (on the tongue) and pyramidal lobe.

92. In thyroidectomy, common complications are damage to the recurrent laryngeal nerve and accidental removal of the parathyroid glands.

93. The fascia of the deep surface of the scalene muscles forms a conical fibrous dome termed the suprapleural membrane (Sibson's fascia) which actually arches over the cupola of the pleura.

94. Lesions of the hypoglossal nerve cause deviation of the tongue when protruded; the deviation occurs to the same side as the lesion because the nerve damage results in lack of function of the genioglossus muscle.

95.   The most common cause of swallowing difficulty is a throat infection.

96.   If food gets impacted in the laryngeal inlet, the vagus can be abruptly stimulated, resulting in cardiac arrest and collapse.

97.   Males are more commonly affected by tongue carcinoma.

98.   The most common sites for tongue cancer are the edges of the tongue.

99.   Tongue carcinoma generally metastasizes very slowly.

100.   Sensitive teeth result from exposure of the tooth dentin (normally, enamel covers the dentin).

101.   When the eustachian tube is blocked, residual air in the tympanic cavity (middle ear) is resorbed, pressure is lowered, a vacuum is created, and the tympanic membrane is retracted; this usually affects hearing.

102.   Swallowing aids in opening the eustachian tube because of the actions of the salpingopharyngeus muscle and the dilator tubae which blends with the tensor veli palatini.

103.   Blood flows freely through the dural sinuses because they have no valves.

104.   Thrombophlebitis of a facial vein can spread to the venous system of the cranium (including cranial veins of the brain) because the facial veins have no valves.

105.   Thrombosis of the cavernous sinus can extend along the retinal vein and produce thrombosis of the retinal vein branches.

106.   Suppurative nasal and sinus infections can lead to thrombophlebitis of the cavernous sinus with subsequent meningitis.

107.   Thrombophlebitis or inflammation of the cavernous sinuses can affect the cranial nerves associated with that sinus: CNs III, IV, VI, and the ophthalmic and maxillary divisions of V (V1 and V2).

108.   The cisterna magna is a site used to obtain CSF samples.

109.   Death involving damage of vital brain structures is usually the result of failure of respiration.

110.   An epidural hemorrhage is an extradural hemorrhage, and is usually caused by a skull fracture.

111.   The bleeding in an epidural hemorrhage occurs between the dura and the periosteum of the calvaria (i.e., outside the dura), and is most often arterial in source.

Boards Boot Camp High-Yield Compendium

112.   The most common site for an epidural hemorrhage-generating skull fracture is the greater wing of the sphenoid (i.e., the "temple"), where the anterior branch of the middle meningeal artery passes through the bone.

113.   Clinically, in an epidural hemorrhage, the patient is knocked unconscious (brief concussion) at injury, then awakens and has a lucid period of several hours (but, sometimes may not), then slips into a coma as the hemorrhage enlarges.

114.   An epidural hemorrhage often also commonly causes a third nerve palsy (as it runs through the superior orbital fissure), resulting in an ipsilateral dilated, fixed pupil due to the hematoma's pressure on the nerve.

115.   Eventually, an epidural hemorrhage may become so large as to cause herniation of the temporal lobe (usually the uncus) through the tentorial incisura near the third nerve origin (third nerve again affected, but at a different site and a later time than that noted in the previous statement/bullet).

116.   A subdural hemorrhage is a bleed between the dura and the arachnoid

117.   A subdural hemorrhage occurs in almost all severe head injuries as a result of stretching and/or tearing of the dura and arachnoid with tearing of the cerebral veins where they enter the superior sagittal sinus. (This, therefore, is a venous bleed).

118.   A subdural bleed may be acute or chronic, with the latter being the result of an unrecognized bleed.

119.   Alcoholics are particularly at risk for subdural hemorrhages due to their proneness to head injuries from falls, alcohol-associated arachnoid edema, and bleeding tendency due to alcoholic liver damage.

120.   The clinical symptoms of a subdural hemorrhage arise 3-6 weeks after the injury and arise when the hemorrhage has organized into a clot; symptoms include headache, confusion, somnolence, and coma.

121.   A subarachnoid hemorrhage is the most common intracranial bleed due to trauma.

122.   Subarachnoid hemorrhage is often associated with cerebral or cerebellar contusion ("bruising") or laceration, resulting in bleeding into the subarachnoid space with concomitant bloody CSF.

123.   Traumatic subarachnoid hemorrhages often occur over the occipital lobes and cerebellum.

124.   Nontraumatic subarachnoid hemorrhages are usually the result of a berry aneurysm rupture along the circle of Willis.

125. In a subarachnoid hemorrhage, the blood in the subarachnoid space acts as an irritant, causing meningeal irritation. The meningeal irritation is manifested by stiff neck, headache, and often loss of consciousness.

126. Other less common causes of subarachnoid hemorrhage are carbon monoxide poisoning, acute cerebral congestion due to status epilepticus, and hemorrhagic diatheses (bleeding disorders).

127. An intracranial hemorrhage is a bleed into the brain substance itself, and is usually arterial in origin.

128. The arteries involved with an intracranial bleed are typically arteries from the circle of Willis or the basal ganglia or internal capsule.

129. Intracranial hemorrhage usually results in paralytic strokes because of the interruption of blood supply to those pathways that transmit signals from the cortex to the brain stem and spinal cord.

130. A cerebral concussion is an abrupt, transient loss of consciousness that follows a hit to the head.

131. A cerebral contusion is bruising to the brain that is visible, and is due to trauma.

132. A cerebral contusion can result in extended loss of consciousness.

133. Gross enlargement (i.e., tumor) of the pituitary gland can place pressure directly onto the internal carotid arteries, giving symptoms of carotid artery occlusion; the tumor may also place pressure directly on the optic chiasma, resulting in bitemporal hemianopsia.

134. A single lesion in the internal capsule can cause a complete unilateral motor and sensory loss.

135. Damage to the cerebellum may result in disturbances of voluntary movement.

136. The blood brain barrier is comprised of the arachnoid barrier layer (which is a blood-CSF barrier) and a true blood-brain barrier comprised of rows of tight junctions between the adjacent endothelial cells of the cerebral capillaries.

137. Nerve cells do not readily reproduce, so any nerve cell damage has serious ramifications.

138. A congenital aneurysm (berry or miliary aneurysm) usually occurs on the circle of Willis, especially at the anterior communicating artery, the middle or anterior cerebral artery, or the basilar artery, all typically at or near an area of bifurcation.

139. Sudden rupture of an aneurysm causes severe dizziness and "the worst headache of my life" due to bleeding into the subarachnoid space; coma may follow a severe hemorrhage.

140. Arteriosclerotic intracranial aneurysms occur either in the vertebral-basilar or internal carotid-cerebral systems.

141. Mycotic aneurysms are due to septic emboli (emboli of microorganisms), and usually occur in the middle or anterior cerebral arteries.

142. A cerebrovascular accident (CVA) is a stroke.

143. A CVA results from a sudden hemorrhage into the brain or an interruption of blood supply leading to brain infarction and tissue death in the area of the brain supplied by the occluded artery.

144. The hemorrhagic type of CVA is usually due to the rupture of an arteriosclerotic artery or aneurysm.

145. A typical site for a hemorrhagic CVA is the lenticulate branch of the middle cerebral artery, resulting in hemorrhage into the basal ganglia and internal capsule.

146. The thrombotic type of CVA is due to thrombosis in an artery to the brain or due an embolus from a distant site; these emboli may be blood clots (usually from the heart – especially think of atrial fibrillation), thrombotic atheromatous material (from fractured or disrupted atheromas), aggregates of platelets (from the walls of medium-sized arteries), or gas bubbles (from large veins opened via trauma or surgery).

147. Hydrocephalus occurs as a result of either overproduction of CSF or inability of CSF to drain from brain.

148. Hydrocephalus causes a rise in CSF pressure resulting in a progressive dilation of the ventricles and ventricular system.

149. There are two types of hydrocephalus: communicating or noncommunicating (obstructive type).

150. The communicating type of hydrocephalus has CSF that is able to move from the lateral ventricle to the lumbar subarachnoid space; it is due to blockage of absorption of CSF in the basilar cisterns or at the pacchionian granulation (as might occur with meningitis and its inflammation of the meninges).

151. The noncommunicating type of hydrocephalus has CSF that is not able to flow from the lateral ventricles to the lumbar subarachnoid space; it is caused by an obstruction in the ventricular system or in the 4th ventricular outflow area.

152. Meningitis may produce a purulent substance in the subarachnoid spaces and cisterns that can cause an obstruction in CSF circulation.

153. A hordoleum is a sty, and is an acute, suppurative inflammation of the gland of Zeiss or Moll (external hordoleum) or a meibomian gland (acute chalazion or internal hordoleum).

154. A chalazion is a chronic granuloma of the eyelid resulting from infection and obstruction of a meibomian gland or its duct.

155. Blepharitis is inflammation of the lid margin, and is due to sebaceous gland infection.

156. Ectropion is eversion of the eyelid; entropion is inversion of the eyelid.

157. Tears are lacrimal gland secretions that are produced when the glands are parasympathetically stimulated via signals from CN VII.

158. Blow-out fractures of the bony margins of the orbit most commonly affect the orbital floor, resulting in herniation of orbital fat into the maxillary sinus.

159. Conjugate movement is the term for when both eyes work together (as they do normally).

160. Paralysis of one or more of the ocular muscles results in diplopia (double vision).

161. The parts of the eye that play a role in refraction (focus of image) are the cornea, the aqueous humor, the crystalline lens, and the vitreous body.

162. Cortical blindness is blindness due to occipital lobe damage.

163. Nearsightedness is myopia, and results when the eyeball it too long and the image focuses in front of the retina.

164. Farsightedness is hyperopia, and results when the eyeball is too short and focus occurs behind the retina.

165. Old sight is presbyopia, and occurs because of lessened ability to accommodate due to a greater difficulty in shaping an increasingly aged lens.

166. Arcus senilis is a benign peripheral corneal degeneration.

167. "Eye grounds" is the term for the fundus of the eye as seen with the ophthalmoscope.

168. The blind spot is the area of the retina where the optic nerve fibers exit the eyeball and retinal vessels enter.

169. The cornea is sensitive to touch and pain and is innervated by the ciliary twigs from the nasociliary nerve (CN V1).

170. An Argyll-Robertson pupil is a pupil that does not constrict for light but that does constrict for near vision, i.e. it does accommodate.

171. An Argyll Robertson pupil is usually caused by a pretectal zone lesion (in the midbrain), the center for light reflexes.

172. Infections or boils in the external auditory canal may cause nausea and vomiting because the general somatic afferent fibers (i.e., pain, sensation) from this area are carried in the vagus nerve which also carries all the parasympathetic fibers to the GI tract (excluding the distal tract).

173. Meniere's Disease produces symptoms of loss of balance and tinnitus; these symptoms are a result of labyrinthal edema and inflammation of the vestibular nerve.

174. CSF rhinorrhea occurs as a result of a fracture to the cribriform plate and tearing of the meninges; a clear fluid (CSF) exudes from the nose.

175. A nosebleed is epistaxis, and typically occurs from the anterior part of the nose in front of the inferior concha; if septal in origin, it generally occurs from "Little's area," an area with a lot of anastomoses.

176. Coccydynia is pain in the coccygeal region and is usually due to separation of the coccyx from the sacrum, often secondary to a fall.

177. Nodose lumbago (rheumatism) is characterized by nodule formation, particularly in the areas of the iliac and sacral crests; it may lead to severe and incapacitating pain.

178. The anterior spinal artery arises from the vertebral arteries; it originates as two small arteries that run downward and fuse into a single vessel, anterior to the medulla at the level of the foramen magnum.

179. There are two posterior spinal arteries, one on each side.

180. There are spinal artery weaknesses: anteriorly at T4 and L1, and posteriorly at T1 and T3. These weaknesses are due to presence of only a few, small radicular arteries in those locations (i.e., there is little supplemental blood flow).

181. The areas of arterial weakness in the spinal arteries are known as the watershed areas of the cord, and are mostly found in the midthoracic region of the cord.

182. Veins from ALL parts of the body interconnect with those around the spinal cord.

183.   The venous plexuses of the spinal cord have incomplete valves or no valves.

184.   Considering #182 and #183, metastases to the spinal cord, particularly from the pelvis, are not uncommon.

185.   If the transverse ligament of the atlas ruptures, the dens may be driven into the cervical portion of the cord resulting in quadriplegia (paralysis of all limbs) or into the medulla resulting in sudden death.

186.   Whiplash (necklash) usually occurs secondary to automobile accidents when the car is struck abruptly from behind. The impact accelerates the car temporarily, and the passenger's torso also moves forward. The free neck and head are thrown violently backward because of their inertia. The neck muscles react to the violent extension, abruptly contracting to cause flexion, but inevitably causing overcompensation by snapping the head forward. The most damage is thought to occur with the abrupt flexion. The cervical injuries may include muscle strain, cervical root damage, subluxation of vertebrae, compression fracture of the vertebrae, and herniation of cervical intervertebral disks.

187.   In the adult, the spinal cord ends at L2. In the neonate, it ends at the lower border of L3.

188.   Spinal punctures are used to withdraw CSF for diagnostic purposes ("spinal tap"), for treatment using antibiotics, and for anesthesia in surgeries involving areas below the thorax.

189.   Extradural injections are used to create anesthesia over a more limited area without the dangers inherent in spinal puncture.

190.   The overlap of peripheral nerves is less extensive in the limbs than it is in the trunk; hence, complete interruption of a single peripheral nerve is typically sensed more in the limbs.

191.   The hand is drained by two sets of veins: the superficial group and the deep group.

192.   Fractures of the clavicle usually occur medially.

193.   The ulna is more subject to fracture due to elbow trauma; the radius is more subject to fracture resulting from falls on hands.

194.   A reverse Colles' fracture is called a Smith's fracture and is usually produced by a fall on the back of the hand while the wrist is flexed.

195.   Most fractures of the carpus (wrist) include the scaphoid bone.

196.   The skin of the palm contains no hair or sebaceous glands, but sweat glands are more numerous (i.e., why one gets the "sweaty" palms).

197.   Dupuytren's contracture is a disorder, often familial, of the palmar aponeurosis. It manifests itself as a progressive fibrosis of the aponeurosis such that one or more digits are pulled into a marked, irreversible flexion at the MCP joint.

198.   The recurrent branch of the median nerve supplies the thenar muscles and is very superficial.

199.   Because of its superficial location, the recurrent branch of the median nerve may be severed by minor lacerations of the palm near the thenar eminence, rendering the thumb nearly useless.

200.   The lumbricals are responsible for placing the fingers into the writing position; the interossei are the muscles responsible for allowing us to type, actively write, and play the piano.

201.   Tenosynovitis is an inflammation of the tendon sheaths that is contained within bursae.

202.   The radial nerve supplies NO muscles in the hand.

203.   As the extensor tendons reach the dorsal aspect of the MCP joint, they expand laterally over the sides of the joints. This expansion of the extensor tendon is referred to as the extensor hood.

204.   The fascia of the finger forms the finger pad (termed the "pulp"); infection of the pulp is called a felon or whitlow.

205.   If breast ducts are invaded by cancer, they may pull and retract, causing invagination of inversion of the nipple.

206.   Shoulder separation (not dislocation) is a dislocation of the acromioclavicular joint, and is a very common injury.

207.   When passing a needle through the thoracic wall as in thoracentesis or paracentesis, it is customary to place the needle close to the upper border of the rib; this is because the vein, artery, and nerve run at the inferior inner aspect of the rib, and run in that order (VAN).

208.   Each bronchopulmonary segment is supplied by its own nerve, artery, and vein.

209.   Each lung has 10 segments. However, the right lung has three lobes while the left lung has only two.

210.   In slightly more than half of cases, the right coronary artery supplies the SA node.

211.   In most cases, the right coronary artery supplies the AV node.

Boards Boot Camp High-Yield Compendium

212.   The term "pericardial sac" refers to both the fibrous layer of the pericardium and parietal layer of serous pericardium. It has a poor blood supply, and expands gradually if the heart enlarges slowly.

213.   The pericardium has two layers: the fibrous layer and the serous layer.

214.   The serous layer of the pericardium has two layers: the visceral pericardium (epicardium; lines the heart) and the parietal pericardium (lines the inner surface of the fibrous pericardium).

215.   The pacemaker of the heart is the sinoatrial node (SA node).

216.   Foreign objects are more likely to enter the right bronchus because the right bronchus is larger and has a less sharp angle than the left.

217.   The "cardiac orifice" of the stomach lies behind the 7th costal cartilage.

218.   The fundus of the gallbladder lies just behind the 9th right costal cartilage.

219.   The veins above the umbilicus anastomoses with those directly below it and with the thoracoepigastric vein; they also communicate with the paraumbilical venous plexus which connects to the portal vein.

220.   Because the superficial epigastric veins at the umbilicus are connected with the portal system, these veins become engorged whenever there is obstruction of the portal system or the inferior vena cava, resulting in caput medusa.

221.   Bleeding peptic ulcers are usually located in the posterior stomach while perforating types of peptic ulcers are usually located anteriorly.

222.   Cancer of the stomach as well as most other GI organs produces metastases in the liver because venous drainage is by way of the portal vein.

223.   Most duodenal ulcers are near the pylorus.

224.   The first part of the duodenum has the poorest blood supply because it is NOT supplied by the arcades, but rather by small branches of the gastroduodenal artery.

225.   The gallbladder is prone to recurrent bacterial infections which are painful (initially felt in the epigastrium).

226.   Because of its tremendous vascularity, the liver is a common site for secondary carcinoma from nearly anywhere in the body (and particularly from the GI tract).

227.   Hepatomegaly is usually associated with one or more of the following disorders: carcinoma, heart failure, fatty infiltration (i.e., as in liver failure), or Hodgkin's disease.

705

228. Portal obstruction will result in engorgement of the veins supplying the portal system, namely causing esophageal varices, hemorrhoids, and caput medusae.

229. A common cause of portal hypertension is liver cirrhosis (the fibrotic bands prevent good venous flow). Other causes of portal hypertension include Budd-Chiari syndrome, portal vein thrombosis, and CHF.

230. ANY degree of spleen enlargement is abnormal

231. Obstruction of the ureter at any level causes ureteral dilation of the parts superior to the obstruction, including dilation of the renal pelvis and calices, resulting in hydronephrosis.

232. The cisterna chyli is located in front of the second lumbar vertebra.

233. A hiatal hernia is an opening, usually located on the left side, of the diaphragm near the esophageal hiatus that permits the abdominal viscera to ascend into the thorax.

234. Spinal cord damage above the sacral region often spares the micturition reflex, but conscious control over onset and duration is lost.

235. The micturition reflex is normally controlled by voluntary contraction of the urethral sphincter (a voluntary, striated muscle) and signals from the cerebral cortex and brainstem via corticospinal tracts to S2,3,4 cord segments.

236. It is the median lobe of the prostate that is important for BPH; enlargement of its mucous glands cause urethral obstruction and adenomas in this lobe are frequent.

237. The anal canal has 4 important landmarks: the anocutaneous line that marks the distal end of the GI tract. Hilton's white line that demarcates the interval between the external and internal and sphincters. The pectin line is the mucocutaneous junction (also known as the pectinate or dentate line), with internal hemorrhoids developing above it and external hemorrhoids developing below it. The anorectal line is the line above the anal crypts and sinuses, and marks the beginning of the anal canal.

238. The pectinate line marks the change from columnar or cuboidal epithelium to the stratified epithelium of the lower part of the canal; this line is important because carcinomas from the two types of epithelium differ.

239. Innervation above the pectinate line is carried afferently through fibers of the pelvis plexus (visceral type); innervation below the line is via somatic nerve fibers in the pudendal nerve.

240. Hemorrhoids are also known as piles.

241.   As the rectum fills with fecal material, parasympathetic stimulation causes it to contract and causes the internal anal sphincter (which is the circular muscle of the intestine in that area) to relax. Once the rectum is filled to about 25% of its capacity, the urge to defecate begins. However, defecation is not permitted because the external anal sphincter, comprised of slips of muscle from the pelvis, remain tonically contracted. When defecation is desired, the external anal sphincter is voluntarily relaxed through motor neuron stimulation. In response, the smooth muscle of the rectum contracts (parasympathetic stimulation), and the feces exit the body. Infra-abdominal pressure also aids in the defection process, such that voluntary contraction of the abdominal muscles while expiring against a closed glottis (Valsalva maneuver) causes pressures in the rectal region.

242.   The ovary is divided into an outer cortex and an inner medulla.

243.   The outer ovarian cortex consists of cellular connective tissue stroma, ovarian follicles, and a surface of a single layer of cuboidal epithelial cells ("simple cuboidal surface epithelium"; germinal epithelium).

244.   The medulla of the ovary consists of loose connective tissue, blood vessels, lymphatics, nerves, some smooth muscle, and a few vestigial tubular structures known as rete ovarii.

245.   An ovarian follicle consists of a developing ovum around which is follicle cells and connective tissue.

246.   Follicles develop while the female is an embryo herself.

247.   While the female is an embryo herself, her primordial sex cells develop into oogonia, which then differentiate into primary oocytes; these primary oocytes develop through prophase of the first meiotic division, after which they enter an arrested dictyotene stage. (Remember, prophase, then metaphase, then anaphase, then telophase). At puberty, the hypothalamus begins to produce gonadotropin-releasing hormone (GnRH). The hormone stimulates FSH (follicle stimulating hormone) release by the anterior pituitary gland. FSH causes the arrested primary oocytes to develop. Some primary oocytes (not all!) emerge from the arrested dictyotene stage and fully complete all of the stages of the first meiotic division. At the same time, the follicle cells surrounding these individual developing oocytes enlarge and proliferate, forming a stratified (many layered) cuboidal epithelium around the oocyte – once this is completed the primary oocyte is now termed a primary follicle. The follicle continues to enlarge, and spaces between follicle cells unite to form one large space; that space is known as the antrum and becomes filled with a fluid know as liquor folliculi. With the formation of the fluid filled antrum, the primary follicle is now known as a secondary (vesicular) follicle. Differentiation of the follicular cells occurs such that the follicular cells around the antrum form a stratified (many-layered) epithelial membrane granulosa that is positioned on a basal lamina. Concurrently, this all becomes surrounded by an inner theca interna which is richly vascularized and an outer theca externa which is very fibrous. The theca interna cells produce androstenedione when stimulated to do so by LH. The androstenedione (a type of androgen) is converted to estrogen by

granulosa cells (remember, granulosa cells surround the antrum) when the latter are stimulated by FSH. The oocyte itself is surrounded by a protein-polysaccharide layer termed the zona pellucida; closely surrounding this are the follicular cells that have developed to form a layer called the corona radiata. The combined oocyte, zona pellucida, and corona radiata project into the antrum of the follicle and are termed the cumulus oophorus.

248.   The fallopian tubes (uterine tubes; oviducts) have four regions: infundibulum, ampulla, isthmus, and interstitial (intramural) portion. The wall of each is comprised of the mucosa, muscularis, and serosa.

249.   The uterus is comprised of, from cephalad to caudad, the fundus, body, and cervix. The body and fundus have three layers: perimetrium (serosa), myometrium (muscularis), and endometrium (mucosa). The perimetrium is the serosal continuation of the broad ligament. The myometrium is comprised of smooth muscle.

250.   The uterine cervix consists of an inner mucosa, a middle muscularis, and an outer adventitia.

251.   The testis is ovoid in shape and surrounded by a thick connective tissue capsule called the tunica albuginea.

252.   The tunica albuginea of the testis sends radiating branches into the substance of the testis, dividing the testis into lobules.

253.   Within the lobules of the testis are seminiferous tubules and loose connective tissue stroma. The stroma contains interstitial cells of Leydig.

254.   Leydig cells are stimulated by LH (luteinizing hormone; in the male, also known as interstitial cell-stimulating hormone (ICSH)) to produce testosterone.

255.   The seminiferous tubules join in groups to form the straight tubules. The straight tubules converge on the rete testis.

256.   The seminiferous epithelium contains additional cells known as Sertoli cells and sex cells in various stages of spermatogenesis.

257.   Sertoli cells are closely joined against one another. They support, protect, and nurture the sex cells. The sex cells are located between the Sertoli cells, and are "blanketed" by them.

258.   Sertoli cells are stimulated by FSH to produce androgen-binding protein which serves to concentrate testosterone for spermatogenesis. They also secrete inhibin.

259.   The bile passages include the gallbladder, the cystic duct, the hepatic ducts, and the common bile duct.

260.   The pancreas is retroperitoneal (except for the tail).

261. The kidneys are completely retroperitoneal.

262. The peritoneal cavity is comprised of the greater and lesser peritoneal sacs.

263. The lesser peritoneal sac (omental bursa) is posterior to the lesser omentum, the caudate lobe of the liver, and the stomach.

264. The greater sac is all of the peritoneal cavity that is not the lesser sac.

265. The greater and lesser sacs of the peritoneal cavity are connected only through the epiploic foramen (of Winslow), which is very small. The anterior border of this opening is formed by the lesser omentum (which here is formed by the hepatoduodenal ligament, and contains the common bile duct, the portal vein, the proper hepatic artery, and the lymphatics and nerves).

266. Indirect inguinal hernia follows the course of the testes during development (therefore, passes through the inguinal canal via the internal opening).

267. Direct inguinal hernias pass through Hesselbach's triangle (the triangle borders = lateral border of the rectus abdominus, the inferior epigastric vessels, and inguinal ligament).

268. There are usually three layers to blood vessels (not capillaries!) and lymphatics: tunica intima (inner layer; endothelium), tunica media (middle layer), and tunica adventitia (outer layer). Capillaries only have an endothelium lining about which is the basal lamina for those endothelial cells, about which are pericytes and some connective tissue.

269. The tunica media is more pronounced in arteries than in veins. All medias contain smooth muscle with varying degrees of elastic fibers, with large arteries such as the aorta having more elastic fibers.

270. The ureter passes anterior to the SI joint and medial to the internal iliac artery.

271. In the male, the ureter passes posterior and inferior to the ductus deferens. In the female, the ureter passes inferior to the uterine artery and lateral to the cervix.

272. The vasa vasorum are small blood vessels that nourish the walls of large vessels.

273. It is the peripheral group of glands (posterior lobe) within the prostate that is important clinically for prostate cancer. When palpated with digital rectal exam, it feels enlarged and "rock hard."

709

274. The ureter passes under the uterine artery. The uterine artery is the "bridge" over the "water" of the ureter – this is an important relationship to remember during any gynecologic surgery.

275. The recurrent laryngeal nerve is vulnerable to injury during thyroidectomy, carotid endarterectomy, and other surgery in that area. Crushing and/or cutting of the nerve transforms the voice to only a whisper.

276. The recurrent laryngeal nerve is a branch of the vagus nerve, and supplies all intrinsic muscles of the larynx, except for the cricothyroid muscle.

277. Pressure on the optic chiasm, like what could happen with a pituitary tumor, results in loss of conduction of certain visual input, causing a bitemporal heteronymous hemianopsia (e.g., loss of vision nearer the temples than the nose (so it is lateral loss in both eyes; "bitemporal") + loss of different visual fields in each eye (e.g., the right side of the right eye visual field and the left side of the left eye visual field; "heteronymous") + loss of an entire ½ of the visual field in each eye ("hemianopsia").

278. Levator palpebrae superioris = a thick muscle that fans out into a wide aponeurosis that inserts into the skin of the upper eyelid; raises lid and is innervated by CN III.

279. Muller's muscle = superior tarsal muscle = the inferior part of the aforementioned aponeurosis and contains SMOOTH muscle fibers. It receives its innervation from sympathetics (which run with CN III).

280. Tarsal glands are positioned deep to the superior tarsal muscle.

281. Horner's syndrome is due to compression of the cervical sympathetic chain by neck injuries, neck tumors, or Pancoast tumors of the lung. This compression INHIBITS sympathetic stimulation of the head ipsilaterally.

282. The sympathetics via the sympathetic plexus (which receives its innervation from the cervical sympathetic chain and rides with CN III) provides innervation and stimulation to the dilator pupillae to permit mydriasis.

283. All tongue muscles are innervated by CN XII (hypoglossal nerve). The muscles of the tongue include the genioglossus (aids in protrusion and depression; when paralyzed, allows the tongue to fall back and obstruct airway), the styloglossus (retracts and curls it up on sides), the hypoglossal (depresses and retrudes), and palatoglossus (elevates the posterior part of the tongue) → and is innervated by CN X and so is typically NOT considered a classis tongue muscle!!!.

284. When there is damage to the CN XII unilaterally (e.g., CVA), the genioglossus that is still being innervated works to protrude the tongue toward the damaged side.

285.   Sensation to the anterior 2/3 of the tongue is conducted by CN VII (specifically the chorda tympani) for taste and by CN V3 (specifically the lingual nerve) for touch and temperature.

286.   Sensation to the posterior 1/3 of the tongue is conducted via CN IX (via the lingual nerve) for taste and via CN IX (via lingual branches) for touch and temperature.

287.   The only mandibular muscle to work in opening the jaw is the lateral pterygoid. The medial pterygoids, masseter, and temporalis all work to close the jaw. All of the muscles in this paragraph are derived from the 1st branchial arch and, therefore, are innervated by CN V (mandibular; V3).

288.   The ONLY abductors of the vocal cords are the posterior cricoarytenoids.

289.   Everything in the larynx is innervated by the recurrent laryngeal nerve EXCEPT for the cricothyroid which is innervated by the external laryngeal nerve.

290.   ALL sensation above the glottis is provided by the internal laryngeal nerve (a branch of the superior laryngeal nerve).

291.   The branches coming off the aorta, in descending order from the diaphragm, are: 1) celiac trunk, 2) superior mesenteric artery, 3) the renal arteries, 4) the testicular or ovarian arteries, 5) the inferior mesenteric artery...and then the aorta splits into the right and left common iliac arteries (and a small branch descends from the split, and is termed the median sacral artery). The first branch off of each common iliac artery is the internal iliac artery.

292.   The celiac trunk splits to become, primarily, the splenic artery and the hepatic artery. A branch that peels off of the hepatic artery is the gastroduodenal artery.

293.   The 3rd part (last part) of the duodenum actually sits between the superior mesenteric artery and the aorta. Just superior to the duodenum, sitting in that crevice with it, is the left renal vein.

294.   The inferior mesenteric artery becomes the superior left colic artery and the superior rectal artery. Branches off of the superior rectal and left colic arteries collectively become the inferior left colic arteries.

295.   Transient ischemic attacks (TIAs) usually begin suddenly and last 2-30 minutes or more (seldom>1-2 hours) then abate without persistent neurologic abnormalities (unlike CVAs which do not abate).

Boards Boot Camp High-Yield Compendium

296. Where's the lesion in a CVA or TIA? Lesions involving the internal carotid artery (which becomes the anterior and middle cerebral arteries) produce unilateral symptoms, contralateral paresis, contralateral sensory loss, or language disturbance. Lesions of the vertebrobasilar system (vertebral artery/basilar artery source) produce either unilateral or bilateral problems (usually bilateral – but not bilateral in same parts of body like spinal cord lesions) with, commonly, any one or more of the following: vertigo, ataxia, diplopia, facial problems (contralateral to torso and limb problems), nausea, confusion, binocular blindness.

297. Wolffian duct = mesonephric duct → remain in male and connect directly to the gonads. Mullerian duct = paramesonephric duct → suppressed in development by MIF (Mullerian inhibiting factor) produced by Sertoli cells; hence, remains undeveloped as the appendix of the testes in males. But, becomes the uterus and fallopian tubes of females!

298. Merkel cells are in the skin, and sense light pressure.

299. Meissner's corpuscles are also known as tactile corpuscles. They are in the skin, being in highest concentration on the fingers and lips, and detect light touch, plus have the highest sensitivity to sensing frequency vibration.

300. Pacinian corpuscles are also known as lamellar corpuscles. They are in the skin and sense vibration and pressure.

301. Free nerve endings are critical in the sensation of pain and temperature. Strangely, at temperatures in excess of 120 degrees F, cold fibers begin to fire again, firing with pain fibers. The patient senses pain and cold, despite the extreme heat.

Disease/Organism	Drug of Choice	Mechanism of Action	Major Side Effects
African sleeping sickness (encephalitic stage; late stage)	Melarsoprol (east) or Eflornithine (west)	Mel: Reacts with sulfhydryl groups, rendering enzymes non-functional Efl: Inhibits ornithine decarboxylase	Mel: Hyper-sensitivity reactions, GI problems, potentially fatal neurotoxicity Efl: Thrombo-cytopenia, seizures
Amoebiasis	Metronidazole	DNA and protein destructive agent	Disulfiram-like reaction with alcohol and darkens urine
Anaerobic infections above the diaphragm	Empirically: Clindamycin	Protein synthesis inhibitor	Strong promotion of C. diff overgrowth
Anaerobic infections below the diaphragm	Empirically: Metronidazole	DNA and protein destructive agent	Disulfiram-like reaction with alcohol and darkens urine
Ankylosing spondylitis	Indomethacin	Inhibits cyclooxygenase, thereby preventing prostaglandin synthesis	Gastric irritation and bleeding, possible perforation
Anthrax	Penicillin (but ONLY after it has been demonstrated to be sensitive to this)	Cell wall synthesis inhibitor	Hypersensitivity reaction

Anxiety Disorder	SSRI or TCA daily, + benzodiazepines as needed	Selective Serotonin Reuptake Inhibitor: blocks the reuptake of serotonin Tricyclic amines: block reuptake of NE and sero-tonin, + block muscarinic, alpha, and histaminic (H1) receptors Benzos: Benzodiaze-pine receptor agonist, causing aug-mented binding of GABA to GABA receptors that results in increased chloride entry into neurons and sub-sequent neuronal inhibition	SSRI: Loss of libido, weight gain, seizure with overdose TCAs: Dry mouth, constipation, urinary retention, weight gain Benzos: Drowsiness, confusion, respiratory depression
Aspergillosis	Voriconazole or Amphotericin B *(vori is preferred)*	Ergosterol synthesis inhibitor (vori) OR Ergosterol antagonist + cell membrane pore former (allows electrolytes to pass freely across cell membrane) (amp B)	Vori: Severe skin reactions, severe hepatotoxicity, transient visual change, and photosensitivity Amp B: Severe nephrotoxicity and ototxicity (amp B)

Asthma	The exact drugs of choice depend upon the classification of asthma, but ALL classifications include among their drugs of choice short-acting beta-two agonists, most especially albuterol	Stimulates beta-2 receptors to cause bronchodilation	Tachycardia
Autoimmune disorders	Steroids, in most cases	Have many anti-inflammatory effects, including decreased prostaglandin synthesis, decreased T cell production, decreased antibody production, decreased capillary permeability	Fat redistribution to central body regions, risk of infections, psychiatric disturbance
Bacillus cereus	Vancomycin or clindamycin	Cell wall and membrane synthesis inhibitor or protein synthesis inhibitor, respectively	Vanco: Red man syndrome Clinda: Strong promotion for C. diff overgrowth
Bacterial vaginosis	Metronidazole	DNA and protein destructive agent	disulfiram-like reaction with alcohol and darkens urine

Boards Boot Camp High-Yield Compendium

Benign Prostatic Hypertrophy (BPH)	5-alpha reductase inhibitors (e.g., finasteride, dutasteride, turosteride)	Inhibits 5-alpha reductase, the enzyme that normally plays a role in the conversion of testosterone to dihydro-testosterone (DHT); such inhibition results in decreased androgenic stimulation to the prostate gland	Erectile dysfunction, decreased libido, and decreased ejaculatory volume
Bipolar disorder	Lithium (although there are many other suitable drugs, and monotherapy is not supported – so a mood stabilizer must be added to another mood stabilizer or to an atypical antipsychotic)	Interferes with normal sodium ion movement and exchange	Ataxia, diabetes insipidus, seizures
Blastomycosis	Itraconazole	Ergosterol synthesis inhibitor	Severe hepatotoxicity
Campylobacter jejuni	Azithromycin *(alternate: erythromycin)*	Protein synthesis inhibitor	QT prolongation and torsade de point
Candidiasis, systemic	Fluconazole	Ergosterol synthesis inhibitor	Hepatotoxicity
Chagas disease (early stage)	Nifurtimox or benznidazole	Destroyer of enzymes via creation of radical oxygen species	Both: abdominal pain, nausea, and vomiting; Nif: exacerbates G6PD deficiency Benz: possibly teratogenic
Chlamydia trachomatis	Doxycycline (plus ceftriaxone to treat presumed gonorrhea, unless ruled out by NAAT)	Doxy: Protein synthesis inhibitor Ceftriaxone: Cell wall synthesis inhibitor	Doxy: staining of children's teeth, photosensitivity, pseudotumor cerebri Ceftriaxone: hypersensitivity

Cholecystitis	Piperacillin + tazobactam	Pip: cell wall synthesis inhibitor Tazo: beta-lactamase inhibitor, thereby preventing destruction of piperacillin by lactamases	Hypersensitivity reactions
Chronic obstructive pulmonary disease (COPD)	Albuterol	Beta-2 agonist	Palpitations
CMV retinitis	Ganciclovir + valganciclovir	DNA synthesis inhibitors	Bone marrow suppression that can lead to aplastic anemia
Congestive heart failure	Digoxin

(for non-exacerbated CHF, typically beta-blockers + ACE inhibitors or ARBs + loop diuretics (or thiazides occasionally) are added to increase longevity, although the digoxin itself is THE treatment for the CHF and resulting inadequate cardiac output) | Inhibits Na/K pump, causing an increase in calcium entry which then causes increased force of contraction and cardiac output | Visual change, arrhythmias |
Conjunctivitis, bacterial (non-GC, non-Chlam)	Fluoroquinolone eye drops	Topoisomerase inhibitor	Mild discomfort
Conjunctivitis, viral	No Rx or chilled artificial tears	Soothes discomfort	N/A
Cryptococcal meningitis	Amphotericin B + flucytosine	Ergosterol antagonist + cell membrane pore former (allows electrolytes to pass freely across cell membrane) + DNA synthesis inhibitor	Amp B: Severe nephrotoxicity and otoxicity Flucytosine: Bone marrow toxicity

717

Diabetes mellitus, Type I	Insulin	Facilitates glucose uptake into fat and skeletal muscle tissue	Hypoglycemia
Diabetes mellitus, Type II	Metformin (as first-line)	Inhibits absorption of glucose from bowel, decreases gluconeogenesis, and increases glucose uptake in fat and skeletal muscle tissue	Adverse reaction with IV contrast agents
Diarrhea, severe	Ciprofloxacin or levofloxacin + metronidazole	Topoisomerase inhibitor + DNA and protein destructive agent, respectively	Cipro and levo: Cartilage damage in children; tendon rupture in the elderly; photosensitivity and CNS toxicity Metronidazole: disulfiram-like reaction with alcohol and darkens urine
Diphtheria	Erythromycin + antitoxin	Protein synthesis inhibitor	QT prolongation and torsade de point
Diverticulitis	Metronidazole and ciprofloxacin	DNA and protein destructive agent + topoisomerase inhibitor, respectively	Metro: disulfiram-like reaction with alcohol and darkens urine Cipro: cartilage damage in children; tendon rupture in the elderly; photosensitivity and CNS toxicity
DVT (deep vein thrombosis)	Heparin	By activating antithrombin, works to inhibit factors II, IX, X, XI, and XII; an anticoagulant	Hemorrhage, hypersensitivity reaction
Encephalitis	Empirically until CSF results return: acyclovir	Viral DNA synthesis inhibitor	Nausea

Boards Boot Camp High-Yield Compendium

Enterobius vermicularis	Mebendazole	Prevent s microtubule formation, preventing microtubule-mediated glucose uptake by organism	Mebendazole: teratogenicity
Erectile Dysfunction	PDE-5 inhibitors	Inhibit phospho-diesterase type 5, thus decreasing the degradation of cyclic GMP in the smooth muscle cells lining the blood vessels supplying the corpus cavernosum of the penis and allowing for smooth muscle relaxation	Priapism, blindness, deafness
Fungal infections, dematiaceous (black molds)	Itraconazole	Ergosterol synthesis inhibitor	Severe hepatotoxicity
Fusarium spp.	Amphotericin B	Ergosterol antagonist + cell membrane pore former (allows electrolytes to pass freely across cell membrane)	Severe nephrotoxicity and ototoxicity
Genital herpes	Acyclovir	DNA synthesis inhibitor	Nausea
Giardiasis	Tinidazole or nitazoxanide	Tin: DNA and protein destructive agent Nit: Inhibits electron transport mechanism, so no ATP is produced	Tin: Disulfiram-like reaction with alcohol Nit: Gi disturbance
Gonorrhea	Ceftriaxone (but standard of practice requires using this drug of choice PLUS doxycycline)	Cell wall synthesis inhibitor + protein synthesis inhibitor, respectively	Ceftriaxone: hypersensitivity reaction Doxycycline: staining of children's teeth, photosensitivity, pseudotumor cerebri

719

Gout	Colchicine (although this is the drug of choice, the first-line drugs (one to be used first) are NSAIDS)	Binds tubulin, preventing WBC migration, proliferation, and release of inflammatory agents	Teratogenic
Hemophilus influenzae	Cefotaxime or ceftriaxone (for life-threatening infection) or amoxicillin-clavulanate (for non-life threatening infection)	Cell wall synthesis inhibitors	Hypersensitivity reaction
Herpes keratitis	Trifluridine eye drops	DNA synthesis inhibitor	Mild irritation
Histoplasmosis	Itraconazole	Ergosterol synthesis inhibitor	Severe hepatotoxicity

HIV (when treatment initiation criteria are met)	ART: 2 NRTI + (1 NNRTI or 1 PI or 1 INTI or 1 CCRA) *Specific combinations that are recommended are:* efavirenz + tenofovir + emtricitabine -or- ritonavir-boosted atazanavir + tenofovir + emtricitabine -or- ritonavir-boosted darunavir + tenofovir + emtricitabine -or- raltegravir + tenofovir + emtricitabine	NRTI (nucleoside reverse transcriptase inhibitor): prevents DNA manufacture from viral RNA by acting as a nucleoside analog NNRTI (non-nucleoside reverse transcriptase inhibitor): prevents DNA manufacture from viral RNA by inhibiting reverse transcriptase PI (protease inhibitor): prevents the cleavage and consequent activation of the major viral protein product in cells, prohibiting viral particle synthesis INTI (integrase inhibitor): inhibits HIV viral integrase, thereby preventing integration and insertion of HIV DNA into human DNA CCRA (CCR5 antagonist): blocks CCR5 receptors on WBCs, blocking viral binding to cell	Numerous, and differ by specific drug within each class
Hypercholesterolemia	HMG CoA reductase inhibitors (statins) or bile acid sequestrants (in reality, the latter are rarely used because of their weak action)	HMG CoA reductase inhibitor: inhibit the enzyme responsible for the rate controlling step of cholesterol synthesis, HMG CoA reductase Bile acid sequestrants: bind cholesterol in bowel and drag it out in stool	Statins: hepatotoxicity, myopathy, rhabdomyolysis Bile acid sequestrants: severe constipation

Boards Boot Camp High-Yield Compendium

Hypertension (except for those with a high coronary artery risk, a history of stable angina, unstable angina, or MI, or those with CHF)	Thiazides	Block sodium uptake at the distal convoluted tubule, causing the sodium and water that "follows" it to be diuresed; although the diuretic effect diminishes with time, the decreased vascular resistance does not	Hypokalemia, hypercalcemia, hyperuricemia, sulfa-allergy
Hyperthyroidism	Radioablation with sodium iodine Alternate is with pharmaco-therapy: beta-blocker + (methi-mazole OR propylthiouracil)	Radioactive iodine: accumulates in thyroid gland, and destroys thyroid tissue Beta-blocker: via beta-1 one blockade, decreases heart rate and force of contraction Methimazole: Inhibits thyroperoxidase, thus blocking iodine addition to thyroglobulin (and this blocks T4 production) Propylthiouracil: inhibits thyroperoxidase (like methimazole) + inhibits 5'-deiodinase, an enzyme necessary for the conversion of T4 to T3	Radioactive iodine: DNA damage via radiation exposure (and the inconvenience of, after treatment, having to abstain from sex for 1 month, from getting pregnant for 6 months), and risk of radiation exposure to household members via toilets, sinks, sheets, clothing, and bare feet Beta-blocker:broncho-constriction, bradycardia, hypotension, erectile dysfunction Methimazole:life-threatening neutropenia, dizziness, nausea-vomiting, pruritis, teratogenic (avoid in 1st trimester pregnancy). Propylthiouracil: nausea-vomiting, pruritis, life-threatening neutropenia, thrombocytopenia, and sudden without-warning fulminant hepatitis resulting in death.

Hypothyroidism	L-thyroxine (levothyroxine)	Synthetic T4 (thyroid hormone)	Palpitations, weight loss, insomnia
Influenza	Oseltamivir or zanamivir	Neuraminidase inhibitor	Zanamivir: bronchospasm Oseltamivir and zanamivir: GI disturbance and neuropsychiatric events
Listeriosis	Ampicillin + gentamicin	Amp: Cell wall synthesis inhibitor Gent: Protein synthesis inhibitor	Amp: Hypersensitivity reaction Gent: Ototoxicity, nephrotoxicity, neurotoxicity
Lyme disease	Doxycycline	Protein synthesis inhibitor	staining of children's teeth, photosensitivity, pseudotumor cerebri
Major depressive disorder	SSRI	Selective Serotonin Reuptake Inhibitor: blocks the reuptake of serotonin	Loss of libido, weight gain, seizure with overdose
Measles	Vitamin A (peds) OR Ribavirin (adults)	VitA: Epithelial cell protection and restoration Rib: Viral transcription inhibitor	VitA: Vitamin A toxicity possible Rib: nausea
Meningitis	Empirically, adult: (ceftriaxone or cefotaxime) + dexamethasone + vancomycin	Cell wall synthesis inhibitor + anti-inflammatory + cell wall and cell membrane synthesis inhibitor, respectively	Hypersensitivity reaction, hyperglycemia, and red man syndrome, respectively
Meningitis prophylaxis of close contacts	For both N. meningitidis and H. influenzae: rifampin	RNA synthesis inhibitor (transcription inhibitor)	Hepatotoxicity and bone marrow suppression
Meningococcal meningitis	Penicillin G	Cell wall synthesis inhibitor	Hypersensitivity reaction

Boards Boot Camp High-Yield Compendium

| MI, acute | Aspirin + heparin + beta-blocker + nitroglycerin + morphine + oxygen | Aspirin: platelet aggregation inhibitor
Heparin: anticoagulant, inhibiting factors II, IX, X, XI, XII
Beta-blocker: via beta-one blockade, decreases heart rate and work of heart, decreasing myocardial oxygen demand
Nitroglycerin: primary – venodilation, decreasing preload and so reducing the work of the heart. Secondary (at higher doses) – arterial dilation, yielding coronary vessel dilation and systemic vasodilation; the latter allows for decreased afterload and consequent reduced work of heart
Morphine: venodilation to decrease preload and work of heart + analgesic to control pain and decrease likelihood for tachycardia (and increased heart work) + anti-anxiety to decrease likelihood for tachycardia (and increased heart work)
Oxygen | Aspirin: hemorrhage, hypersensitivity
Heparin: hemorrhage
Beta-blocker: broncho-constriction, hypotension, bradycardia
Nitroglycerin: hypotension
Morphine: respiratory depression, hypotension |

Mild diarrhea	Loperamide	Decreases pre-stalsis via opioid receptor agonism	Constipation
MRSA	Vancomycin	Cell wall and cell membrane synthesis inhibitor	Red man syndrome (erythema and hypotension)
Myasthenia gravis	Physostigmine or neostigmine	Cholinesterase inhibitors, thereby blocking the enzyme responsible for acetylcholine degradation	Increased bladder and GI motility
Mycoplasma pneumoniae	Azithromycin or doxycycline	Protein synthesis inhibitors	Azith: QT prolongation and torsade de point Dox: staining of children's teeth, photosensitivity, pseudotumor cerebri
Neuropathic pain, diabetic	Pregabalin	Inhibits Ca entry into presynaptic neurons (so inhibits neutrotransmitter release), plus modulates CNS GABA action	Myopathy, rhabdomyolysis, vision changes
Neuropathic pain, non-diabetic	Gabapentin	May mediate GABA metabolism, re-uptake, and release	Sedation
Osteomyelitis	Empirically: Nafcillin or oxacillin	Cell wall and cell membrane synthesis inhibitor	Rash
Osteoporosis	Bis-phosphonates	Osteoclast inhibitor and osteoclast apoptosis inducer	Heartburn, nausea, erosive gastritis, jaw osteonecrosis
Otitis externa	ofloxacin drops or (polymyxin + neomycin + hydrocortisone drops) or other combinations	Oflox: Topo-isomerase inhibitor Polymyx: Disrupts bacterial cell membranes (esp. effective against Pseudomonas) Neomycin: Protein synthesis inhibitor Hydrocortisone: Inhibits inflammation	Hypersensitivity reaction

Pancreatitis	Nothing by mouth, IV fluids, and opioids for pain control	Opioids stimulate opioid sigma receptors to mediate pain control	Opioids: respiratory depression
Parkinson's disease	Dopaminergic agents (e.g., levodopa, pramipexole)	Either are converted to dopamine (e.g., levodopa) or stimulate the dopamine receptor	Impulse control disorders, sleep attacks, hallucinations
PE (pulmonary embolus)	Heparin	By activating antithrombin, works to inhibit factors II, IX, X, XI, and XII; an anticoagulant	Hemorrhage, hypersensitivity reaction
Peptic ulcer	Omeprazole	Proton pump inhibitor	Increased gastric carcinoids
Pneumocystis jiroveci (formerly Pneumocystis carinii)	Trimethoprim-sulfamethox-azole	Folate synthesis/utilization inhibitor	Megaloblastic anemia, nausea
Pneumonia (empirically before cause is known)	(Ceftriaxone or ertapenem) + azithromycin (adult tx)	Cef/Ert: Cell wall synthesis inhibitor Azi: Protein synthesis inhibitor	Cef/Ert:hyper-sensitivity reaction Azi: QT prolong-ation and torsade de pointe
Prostatitis, ≤ 35 years old	Ceftriaxone followed by doxycycline	Cell wall synthesis inhibitor then protein synthesis inhibitor	Ceftriaxone: hypersensitivity reaction Doxycycline: staining of children's teeth, photosensitivity, pseudotumor cerebri
Prostatitis, > 35 years old	Fluoroquinolone or trimethoprim-sulfamethox-azole	Topoisomerase inhibitor or folate utilization/synthesis inhibitor, respectively	Fluoroquinolone: tendon rupture in elderly, CNS- and photo-sensitivity Trimethoprim-sulfa-methoxazole: megaloblastic anemia, nausea
Pseudomembranous Colitis	Metronidazole	DNA and protein destructive agent	disulfiram-like reaction with alcohol and darkens urine

Scedosporium apiospermum	Voriconazole	Ergosterol synthesis inhibitor	Severe skin reactions, severe hepatotoxicity, transient visual change, and photosensitivity
Scedosporium proliferans	Itraconazole	Ergosterol synthesis inhibitor	Severe hepatotoxicity
Seizure, absence	Ethosuximide	Unknown, but may decrease calcium ion movement in thalamus	Nephrotoxicity, hepatotoxicity, grand mal seizure
Seizure, febrile (ongoing ones)	Phenobarbital	Increases GABA effects (an inhibitory neurotransmitter) via inhibition of Na/K transport	Decreased cognitive performance, respiratory depression
Seizure, generalized (tonic-clonic)	Valproic acid	Increases CNS GABA concentration and activity	CNS depression, hepatotoxicity, pancreatitis, life-threatening drug interactions, GI irritation, SIADH, thrombocytopenia, Stevens-Johnson
Seizure, partial	Carbamazepine	Na channel blocker	Bone marrow suppression, aplastic anemia, agranulocytosis, severe skin reactions, cardiac arrhythmias, hepatotoxicity, hypothyroidism
Shigellosis	Azithromycin or any fluoroquinolone	Protein synthesis inhibitor or a topoisomerase inhibitor, respectively	Azithro: QT prolongation and torsade de point Fluoroquinolone: Cartilage damage in children; tendon rupture in the elderly; photosensitivity and CNS toxicity
Sporotrichosis	Itraconazole	Ergosterol synthesis inhibitor	Severe hepatotoxicity
Status epilepticus	Diazepam	Stimulates GABA receptor	Sedation

Boards Boot Camp High-Yield Compendium

Streptococcus pneumoniae	Penicillin G	Cell wall synthesis inhibitor	Hypersensitivity reaction
Streptococcus pyogenes	Penicillin G, V or benzathine PCN	Cell wall synthesis inhibitors	Hypersensitivity reaction
Syphilis	Penicillin G	Cell wall synthesis inhibitor	Hypersensitivity reaction
Thrush	Fluconazole	Ergosterol synthesis inhibitor	Hepatotoxicity
Thyroid storm	Propranolol + acetaminophen + glucocorticoids + propylthiouracil (followed at least 1 hour later with Lugol iodine)	Prop: beta-1 and -2 blockade Aceta: Inhibits COX (antipyretic) Glucocort and PTU: Inhibit T4 conversion to T3 (PTU also inhibits T4 production) Lugol I: Blocks thyroid hormone release	Prop: hypotension, bradycardia, bronchoconstriction Aceta: Stevens-Johnson syndrome Glucocorticords: Hyperglycemia PTU: Liver failure, agranulocytosis Lugol I: Esophageal and gastric lesions
Trichinosis	Albendazole + prednisone	Alb: Prevent microtubule form-ation, preventing microtubule-med-iated glucose uptake by helminth Pred: Inhibits phospholipase A2	Alb: Teratogenic; hepatotoxicity and bone marrow toxicity Pred: Psychiatric disturbance, increased risk of other infections
Trichomoniasis	Metronidazole	DNA and protein destructive agent	Disulfiram-like reaction with EtOH; also darkens urine
Trigeminal neuralgia	Carbamazepine	Na channel blocker	Bone marrow suppression, aplastic anemia, agranulocytosis, severe skin reactions, cardiac arrhythmias, hepatotoxicity, hypothyroidism
UTI, inpatient	Ciprofloxacin or levofloxacin	Topoisomerase inhibitor	Cartilage damage in children, tendon rupture in elderly, photosensitivity
UTI, outpatient	Trimethoprim-sulfamethox-azole	Folate utilization/synthesis inhibitor	Megaloblastic anemia, nausea
Vaginal candidiasis	Miconazole	Ergosterol synthesis inhibitor	Hepatotoxicity, but limited due its topical application

APPENDIX A   BIOCHEMISTRY ADDENDUM

MORE BIOCHEMISTRY FACTS
The following "knowledge vignettes" cover a wide variety of biochemistry topics that, although are not as strongly emphasized on boards as the topics covered in the Biochemistry Section of this book, may appear on questions from time to time and are specifically presented herein because of their history of occasionally being on the exams, more commonly the USMLE.

Proteins are comprised of amino acids that are linked to one another via peptide bonds. Peptide bonds join the alpha-amino group of one amino acid to the alpha-carboxyl group of another amino acid, forming a chain of amino acids known as a polypeptide or a protein.

All amino acids located in human proteins are L-amino acids. D-amino acids are associated with bacterial cell walls and some antibiotics.

Proteins can have a primary structure, a secondary structure, a tertiary structure, and a quaternary structure.

The primary structure is determined simply by the sequence of amino acids comprising that protein.

The secondary structure is determined by the regular or repeating arrangements that can arise when the chain of amino acids doubles back on other amino acids in the chain or interacts with other parts of the chain in a manner to form certain repeating patterns. Examples include alpha-helix, beta-sheets, and beta-bends. These secondary structures, since they represent interactions between amino acids already in the chain, are stabilized by hydrogen bonds.

Tertiary structure is characterized by domains, or special folding and contortions (non-regular) assumed by the protein. These domains are stabilized by hydrophobic interactions, hydrogen bonds, ionic bonds, and disulfide bonds maintained between amino acids that are usually not even beside one another in the chain.

Quaternary structure is the structure of a protein that is comprised of more than one polypeptide, with those separate polypeptides associated with one another. These multi-polypeptide structures are stabilized by non-covalent bonds such as hydrogen bonds, hydrophobic interactions, and ionic bonds.

■■■'

Hemoglobin without oxygen assumes the deoxy form, also known as the taut (T) form. Hemoglobin bound to oxygen is the oxygenated form, also known as the relaxed (R) form. The R form, once created, has a high affinity for binding even more oxygen. Hemoglobin can bind up to 4 oxygen molecules (O_2) at a time. So, the more oxygen that binds, the more affinity hemoglobin has to bind even more, up to a total of 4. This yields a sigmoidal curve (S-shaped) when plotting hemoglobin saturation against available oxygen pressure (pO_2) – this is known as the oxygen-dissociation curve.

The ability of hemoglobin to release its bound oxygen is controlled by 4 main features: pO_2, pH, pCO_2, and 2,3-BPG (bisphosphoglycerate) concentration. Oxygen release is facilitated when the pH is low, when pCO_2 is high, when 2,3-BPG is high (a byproduct of glycolysis), and when pO_2 is low – in other words, all conditions that are present when tissues are metabolically very active and, consequently, likely in need of more oxygen.

Carbon monoxide binds hemoglobin's iron with great affinity, stabilizing the hemoglobin into the R form (therefore, preventing oxygen release from the hemoglobin). *Left shift*

The most common adult hemoglobin is HbA. It is comprised of 2 alpha and 2 beta globin chains. Another less common adult hemoglobin in HbA2. It is comprised of 2 alpha and 2 delta globin chains. Fetal hemoglobin (HbF) is comprised of 2 alpha chains and 2 gamma chains. Notice that alpha globin is always necessary for the manufacture of any type of hemoglobin.

Hemoglobin A1C is glycosylated hemoglobin A, and is formed when high plasma glucose levels are maintained (such as in uncontrolled diabetes mellitus). It provides a convenient measure of chronic glucose levels over the past 120 days (the lifespan of the RBC).

• •

Collagen is protein comprised of a triple helix of alpha polypeptide chains (each alpha chain contains 1000 amino acids). The alpha chains are stabilized in the helical formation together by hydrogen bonds.

Collagen is an extremely important fibrous protein necessary to the structure of tendons, bones, skin, corneas, all cartilage, and blood vessels – as well as the vitreous body of the eye.

The amino acids most important to collagen structure are glycine and proline whereby they form a repeating chain of: glycine + (usually) proline + (usually) hydroxyproline or hydroxylysine. Vitamin C is critical to the manufacture of hydroxylysine and hydroxyproline – that is why scurvy (vitamin C deficiency) results in significant connective tissue pathology.

Enzymes are proteins that catalyze reactions – they, themselves, are unchanged by the reaction.

Some enzymes require cofactors or coenzymes for activity. Cofactors are inorganic substances such as metal ions (e.g., magnesium, iron, etc). Coenzymes are organic substances, such as vitamins.

Competitive inhibitors of enzymes have increased effect with increased concentrations. They complete with the substrate (the substance that normally temporarily binds to the active site of the enzyme to undergo the catalysis for the reaction) for binding at the active site of the enzyme. Their actions are reversible by adding more substrate. They increase the Km without affecting the Vmax of the enzyme. (Km = the substrate concentration at which the reaction velocity is at 50%; Vmax = the maximum reaction velocity).
Noncompetitive inhibitors bind to the enzyme at a site other than the active site. They, therefore, do not compete with the substrate. Their effects are irreversible and independent of substrate concentration. They decrease the enzyme's Vmax, but do not affect the Km.

Isoenzymes are enzymes that catalyze the same reaction; they are also termed isozymes. They are different molecules and, therefore, may not share the same structure – but they do catalyze the same reaction. An example of isozymes is creatine kinase – there is CK-MB (for cardiac muscle), CK-MM (for skeletal muscle), and CK-BB (for brain).

Glucose enters cells by crossing those cells' membranes. This is accomplished via the assistance of membrane-bound glucose transporters – there are at least 14 different types known to exist (they are considered to be isoforms of one another). The most important ones are GLUT-1, GLUT-2, and GLUT-4.

GLUT-1 is the most common glucose transporter of RBC cell membranes and is also an abundant glucose transporter in the cell membranes of the cells of the brain. It is insulin independent, meaning that glucose can enter these tissues at will, without the aid of insulin.

GLUT-2 is in the cell membranes of hepatocytes, renal cells, and pancreatic beta-islet cells. It is insulin independent.

GLUT-4 is found in skeletal muscle and adipose tissue. GLUT-4 transporters are known as the insulin-sensitive glucose transporters. In other words, these transporters are insulin-dependent, meaning that the number of transporters available at a given moment on these cell membranes is directly controlled by

731

the amount of insulin available at that time. Thus, glucose can only effectively enter skeletal muscle and adipose tissue when insulin is present.

Pyruvate is the end-product of glycolysis, the process whereby glucose is metabolized to yield energy in the form of ATP. Pyruvate has 4 possible fates: 1) In cells that lack mitochondria (such as RBCs) or in cells that are deprived of adequate amounts of oxygen (such as during hypoxia, shock, or ischemia, or during vigorous exercise of muscles), pyruvate is converted to lactic acid. Lactate dehydrogenase (LDH) catalyzes this reaction. 2) Via the action of pyruvate dehydrogenase, pyruvate can be converted to acetyl CoA, a major fuel for the citric acid cycle, 3) Pyruvate can be converted to oxaloacetate, a citric acid cycle intermediate, via the enzymatic action of pyruvate carboxylase – this reaction is favored in certain cells when there is glucose deficiency and gluconeogenesis is initiated, 4) In some microorganisms, pyruvate carboxylase works to reduce pyruvate to ethanol.

Lactic
Acid

lactate
dehydrogenase

Pyruvate

pyruvate
dehydrogenase

Acetyl COA

The TCA (tricarboxylic acid) cycle is the citric acid cycle. It is also known as the Krebs cycle. The major fuel for it is acetyl CoA, which is the by-product of enzymatic action of pyruvate dehydrogenase on pyruvate. A potent inhibitor of pyruvate dehydrogenase and, thus, a strong inhibitor of TCA cycle function is arsenic.

Each cycle of the TCA cycle yields 1 ATP (or GTP) + 1 FADH2 + 3 NADH. The NADHs and the FADH go on to be oxidized by the electron transport chain after their manufacture in the TCA cycle; that yields about 11 ATPs from the NADHs and FADH.

....

Glycolysis yields 4 ATPs and 2 NADHs and 2 pyruvates. However, it also uses 2 ATPs. Thus, the net ATP production directly from glycolysis is 2. However, the NADH produced via glycolysis is oxidized aerobically to later, ultimately, result in the manufacture of 3 ATPs per NADH. Furthermore, each pyruvate is metabolized in the TCA cycle to yield 1 ATP and in the electron transport pathway to yield 11 ATPs – and, remember, 2 pyruvates (not 1) are created from 1 glucose molecule that undergoes glycolysis.
>>>

Molecules that can be used for gluconeogenesis (the de novo synthesis of glucose in the body) are gluconeogenesis precursors; they include:
All glycolysis intermediates
All intermediates of the TCA cycle

Lactate (a product of pyruvate metabolism in cells either without mitochondria or cells deprived of oxygen)
Alpha-ketoacids (by-products of the metabolism of "glucogenic" amino acids; these amino acids include alanine, arginine, asparagine, aspartate, cysteine, glutamate, glutamine, glycine, histidine, proline, serine, methionine, and valine, as well as those that are additionally ketogenic: threonine, tyrosine, tryptophan, isoleucine, and phenylalanine)
Glycerol (a product of the hydrolysis of triglycerides (fats))

The primary locations for gluconeogenesis are the kidney and the liver.

For gluconeogenesis, pyruvate is converted to phosphoenolpyruvate (PEP) via the enzymatic actions of PEP carboxykinase and pyruvate carboxylase. PEP carboxykinase controls the rate-limiting step for gluconeogenesis. Its manufacture is increased by glucagon and decreased by insulin.

,,,

The 2 major glycogen storage sites are skeletal muscle and the liver. In skeletal muscle, the glycogen is stored as a glucose reservoir for exercising muscle which needs more glucose than that being supplied by the bloodstream. Glycogen in liver serves as a glucose reserve for the body during times of low serum glucose, such as between meals.

Dietary lipids (e.g., consumed lipids) include mostly cholesterol, cholesterol ester, phospholipids, triglycerides (fats), and fatty acids.

Digestion of fats begins in the mouth with lingual lipase action. It is continued in the stomach by that enzyme plus gastric lipase. In the duodenum, the lipids are emulsified by the action of peristalsis and the detergent-action of bile salts. Emulsification is important to allow for small droplet formation from the lipids, allowing better interaction of these lipids with enzymes and mucosal surfaces. Furthermore, pancreatic enzymes released to the duodenum also help to degrade the lipids. These pancreatic enzymes include pancreatic lipase (digests fats), phospholipase A2 (digests phospholipids), lysophospholipase (digests phospholipids), and cholesterol esterase (digests cholesterol esters to cholesterol). The overall control of pancreatic release of enzymes is maintained by an enzyme known as cholecystokinin (CCK), which is produced by the intestinal mucosa in response to lipids and partially digested proteins. The by-products of lipid digestion form micelles that can cross the brush border of the small intestine. Individual lipids simply enter the cells lining the intestinal lumen. All of these lipids and lipid by-products, along with the fat-soluble vitamins (A, D, E, K), combine with a protein known as apo-B48 (an apoprotein) to form a chylomicron, a type of lipoprotein. This chylomicron is then released to the lymphatic system and eventually delivered to the bloodstream.

Fatty acids are used to manufacture fats (triglycerides). They either come from one's diet or are synthesized de novo in the body. Most de novo synthesis occurs in the liver, using primarily either excess carbohydrate or protein as precursors. These precursors provide acetyl CoA which is used to manufacture fatty acids (as well as many other products). Fatty acid synthesis occurs in the cytoplasm of cells.

The rate-limiting step is controlled by acetyl CoA carboxylase. It is activated by insulin and inhibited by glucagon and epinephrine. The end-product of fatty acid synthesis is palmitoyl CoA. Palmitoyl CoA can be further elongated and modified to create all other fatty acids.

Another site of high fatty acid synthesis is the lactating mammary gland.

For fatty acids to be degraded, they must enter the mitochondrion. The acyl CoA enters the mitochondrion via carnitine palmitoyltransferases I and II. Upon entering the mitochondrion, the acyl CoA undergoes beta-oxidization. Beta-oxidation is the process whereby the fatty acid chain is shortened 2 carbons at a time. That 2-carbon split-off product is acetyl CoA. Hence, the products of fatty acid (acyl CoA) beta-oxidation are acetyl CoA molecules and a lot of ATP. A tremendous amount of ATP is produced because, for each acetyl CoA generated, 1 FADH2 and 1 NADH are produced. The NADH and FADH2 enter the TCA cycle (which is also in the mitochondrial matrix); each NADH yields 3 ATPs and each FADH2 yields 2 ATPs. So, for every 2 carbons removed from the fatty acid chain, 1 acetyl CoA, 1 NADH, and 1 FADH2 is produced. In the TCA cycle, the acetyl CoA yields 1 ATP, the NADH yields 3 ATPs, and the FADH2 yields 2 ATPs. Hence, the longer the fatty acid chain, the greater the energy yield.

If an odd-numbered fatty acid is beta-oxidized, the final product, after multiple 2-carbon sets have been cleaved, is a 3-carbon molecule known as propionyl CoA. Propionyl CoA undergoes a unique reaction that, ultimately, yields succinyl CoA. Vitamin B12 is required for such propionyl CoA metabolism.

Nearly all cells of the human body synthesize cholesterol. Cholesterol is essential for multiple functions:

1) It helps to stabilize all eukaryotic, including human cell, plasma membranes
2) It is the precursor to all steroid hormones (aldosterone, cortisol, androgens, estrogens, and progestins)
3) It is used in the synthesis of bile acids

Cholesterol is synthesized in the cytoplasm from acetyl CoA. The rate-limiting step of cholesterol synthesis is controlled by the enzyme, HMG CoA reductase. Potent activators to this enzyme are insulin as well as low cholesterol levels. It is inhibited by cholesterol and HMG CoA reductase inhibitors (e.g., "statins").

There are 2 mechanisms by which damaged or excess proteins are removed from cells and surrounding areas:
1) Ubiquitin-proteosome mechanism (intracellular proteins that are no longer useful, that are damaged, or that are present in excess quantities are tagged with ubiquitin; this allows for their recognition and eventual destruction by a proteosome)
2) Lysosomal systems (the enzymes of lysosomes degrade extracellular proteins)

The amino groups of all amino acids (except lysine and threonine) are eventually transferred to glutamic acid. The enzymes that catalyze this transfer are aminotransferases, and include ALT (alanine aminotransferase) and AST (aspartate aminotransferase). The co-enzyme for all of these reactions is vitamin B6.

The glutamate can then be deaminated (e.g., the amino group is removed) in the liver via an enzyme termed glutamate dehydrogenase. This yields ammonia.

Glutamate can also be deaminated in tissues other than the liver, again yielding ammonia. This ammonia is transported in the bloodstream to the liver by one of two mechanisms:

1) glutamate and ammonia join to form glutamine
2) pyruvate and ammonia join to form alanine

When the alanine and glutamine arrive at the liver via the bloodstream, they are then degraded by the liver to, once again, liberate the ammonia.

Some of the ammonia in the liver is released to the bloodstream and departs the body via the urine. However, most of it is converted to urea in the liver. This is accomplished via the urea cycle.

The urea cycle is the most important means by which the body has of disposing of nitrogen. The rate-limiting step of the urea cycle is controlled by the enzyme, carbamoyl phosphate synthetase I. This enzyme catalyzes the first step in the process: the combination of carbon dioxide + ammonia + 2 ATPs to form carbamoyl phosphate.

Carbamoyl phosphate joins with ornithine to form citrulline. This step and the one prior to it occur in the mitochondrial matrix. Then, the citrulline is transported to the cytosol where it combines with aspartate to yield arginosuccinate. Arginosuccinate is cleaved to form fumarate and arginine. Arginine then is cleaved to form ornithine (which enters the mitochondrial matrix to interact with newly formed carbamoyl phosphate in order to continue the cycle) as well as, most importantly, urea (a molecule that contains 2 nitrogens destined for excretion).

The urea then diffuses out of the liver and is delivered to the kidneys via the bloodstream.

Patients with severe liver disease are not capable of adequately undertaking the urea cycle; as a result, ammonia is not converted to urea. Clinically, this creates hyperammonemia or high serum ammonia levels. If high enough, it may cause hepatic encephalopathy.

Patients with severe kidney disease are incapable of excreting adequate amounts of urea. Due to the resulting increased serum urea levels, a greater amount of urea is transferred to the intestines (usually only small amounts are transferred to that location). The action of urease, a bacterial enzyme, on the urea produces carbon dioxide and ammonia. The ammonia is largely reabsorbed back into the bloodstream, causing hyperammonemia.

Kidney disease also results in elevated BUN (blood urea nitrogen). The urea nitrogen component of the test is due to serum urea; it is elevated in kidney disease secondary to the kidney's inability to excrete it. High serum urea is termed "azotemia." "Uremia" is the term used to describe the clinical manifestations of severe azotemia.

Accordingly, severe liver disease results in a decreased BUN, secondary to the liver's inability to synthesize urea from ammonia.

The non-essential amino acids are those amino acids that can be synthesized in the human body. Essential amino acids are those amino acids that cannot be synthesized in the human body and that, therefore, must be derived from dietary sources.

The non-essential amino acids are:

Alanine	Arginine	Asparagine	Aspartate	Cysteine	Glutamate
Glutamine	Glycine	Proline	Serine	Tyrosine	

The essential amino acids are:

Methionine	Threonine	Valine	Isoleucine	Leucine
Lysine	Tryptophan	Histidine	Phenylalanine	

Amino acids can also be classified as either glucogenic or ketogenic.

The ketogenic amino acids are those that can form acetoacetate (a ketone body) or one of its precursors (acetyl CoA or acetoacetyl CoA). The only amino acids that are strictly ketogenic are leucine and lysine (which happen to also be essential amino acids!). Tyrosine, Tryptophan, Phenylalanine, Threonine, and Isoleucine are both ketogenic and glucogenic.

Glucogenic amino acids are those whose carbon skeletons can be used in gluconeogenesis. Accordingly, any amino acid that can form any of the intermediates of gluconeogenesis are glucogenic. Such intermediates that amino acids can become include pyruvate (alanine, tryptophan, threonine, serine, glycine, cysteine), acetyl CoA (isoleucine), acetoacetate (phenylalanine, tryptophan, and tyrosine) which then becomes acetyl CoA, oxaloacetate (asparagine, aspartate), alpha-ketoglutarate (glutamate, glutamine, arginine, histidine, and proline), succinyl CoA (isoleucine, methionine, threonine, and valine) and fumarate (phenylalanine and tyrosine).

Purines and pyrimidines are the nitrogen-containing bases that, in conjunction with a pentose monosaccharide (ribose or deoxyribose) and one or more phosphates, forms a nucleotide.

The pyrimidines include cytosine (C), uracil (U), and thymine (T). Purines include adenine (A) and guanine (G).

Pyrimidines are formed from glutamine (an amino acid), aspartate (an amino acid), carbon dioxide, and PRPP (5-phosphoribosyl-1-pyrophosphate, a product of the enzymatic action of PRPP synthetase on ribose-5-phosphate, a 5 carbon sugar).

Purines are formed from glutamine (an amino acid), aspartate (an amino acid), glycine (an amino acid), carbon dioxide, N10-formyl tetrahydrofolic acid, and PRPP (5-phosphoribosyl-1-pyrophosphate, a product of the enzymatic action of PRPP synthetase on ribose-5-phosphate, a 5 carbon sugar).

The committed step in pyrimidine synthesis is controlled by carbamoyl phosphate synthetase II, the enzyme that catalyzes the synthesis of carbamoyl phosphate from glutamine and carbon dioxide. This important step is activated by ATP and PRPP and inhibited by UTP (one end-product of pyrimidine nucleotide synthesis).

The committed step in purine synthesis is controlled by glutamine:phosphoribosyl pyrophosphate amidotransferase, the enzyme that catalyzes the synthesis of 5'-phosphoribosylamine from glutamine and PRPP. This important step is activated by inorganic phosphate and inhibited by purine nucleotide di- and triphosphates (e.g., molecules comprised of 1 purine base + 1 ribose sugar + 2 or 3 phosphates → the end-products of purine nucleotide synthesis).

....

Insulin is synthesized by pancreatic beta-islet cells. Precursors to its manufacture are preproinsulin that then becomes proinsulin. Proinsulin is cleaved to form insulin.

Activators to its release (via exocytosis) into the blood stream are an increase in serum glucose levels, an increase in serum amino acid levels, and secretin, a hormone secreted by the intestinal mucosa in response to a low pH of chyme (e.g., food acidified by the stomach that is passing into the intestine). The most potent of these activators is serum glucose. Inhibitors to its release are epinephrine and sympathetic nervous system activation.

The overall effects of insulin include:

1) increased glucose uptake into skeletal muscle and adipose tissue
2) increased synthesis of proteins
3) increased synthesis of fat
4) increased synthesis of glycogen

It is obvious why it is considered an anabolic (building) hormone.

_____

Glucagon is secreted by pancreatic alpha-islet cells. Activators to its release include decreased serum glucose levels, decreased serum amino acid levels, and epinephrine (and any sympathetic nervous system stimulation). Its release is inhibited by elevated serum glucose levels and insulin.

Glucagon serves to bind to glucagon receptors on the liver. This results in stimulation of adenylyl cyclase which results in the synthesis of cAMP in the liver. The cAMP activates protein kinase which works to stimulate several processes, including glycogenolysis, gluconeogenesis, ketogenesis, and amino acid uptake.

The Fed State is comprised of ingestion of food followed by the absorptive state. The absorptive state is the 2-4 hour period of time following ingestion of food substances. During the absorptive state, there are transient increases in serum glucose, amino acids, and fats (most of which are packaged within chylomicrons). The increased glucose and amino acid levels in the serum result in release of insulin and a decreased release of glucagon. The insulin facilitates glucose uptake into skeletal muscle and adipose tissue, and aids amino acid uptake into most tissues. Tissues not insulin dependent readily take up glucose. As a result, the absorptive state can be said to be an anabolic phase. The liver uses the glucose to synthesize glycogen. The liver, as well as all other tissues, replenish protein needs via utilization of the amino acids they take up. In addition, the chylomicrons deliver triglycerides to skeletal muscle and adipose tissue; and, the remaining chylomicron structure, the "chylomicron remnant," then delivers the rest of its lipids, including any remaining triglycerides, to the liver. The liver, in turn, manufactures triacylglycerols and re-packages any chylomicron-delivered fats into VLDLs (very low density lipoproteins) which serve to either directly or indirectly redistribute all lipids to peripheral tissues. The adipose tissue, now in receipt of fatty acids and fats from chylomicrons (and VLDLs) as well as glucose via the actions of insulin, manufactures and stores more fat. Skeletal muscle, now in receipt of amino acids and glucose, via the actions of insulin, as well as fats

and fatty acids (via delivery from chylomicrons and VLDLs), now synthesizes glycogen and proteins and uses the fatty acid as an immediate fuel source. The brain uses glucose exclusively during the fed state.

The Fasting State, a state developed by the absence of food, is marked by low levels of serum glucose, amino acids, and fats. Insulin secretion is decreased and glucagon release is increased. This is a catabolic period in which the body must catabolize available storage molecules to provide adequate fuel sources. Accordingly, in response to the high glucagon levels, the liver undertakes glycogenolysis and gluconeogenesis, releasing the newly cleaved off or formed glucose to the bloodstream. Also, as a result to decreased insulin levels (and increased sympathetic nervous system tone), hormone sensitive lipase in adipose tissue becomes highly active, resulting in triglyceride hydrolysis and the release of fatty acids and glycerol to the bloodstream. The liver uses these fatty acids by beta-oxidizing them, providing abundant ATP as well as an ample supply of acetyl CoA. This acetyl

CoA is then converted to ketone bodies which are subsequently released to the bloodstream. The brain is able to, in the fasting state, use both glucose and ketone bodies as a fuel source. Muscle use the fatty acids released by adipose tissue, glucose from it glycogen stores, and its own amino acids from the degradation of its own structural proteins as a fuel source.

It should be noted that resting muscle in the fed state uses fatty acid as its fuel source. And, exercising muscle in the fed state undertakes glycogenolysis to gain glucose as an additional fuel source. And, in fact, during extreme exercise, the glucose-6-phosphate produced in excess via glycogenolysis in skeletal muscle is converted to lactate via anaerobic processes. In the fasting state, as glycogen stores are depleted, fatty acids become the primary fuel source. Ketone bodies are used also. After about 3 weeks of fasting, muscle virtually ceases using ketone bodies and relies almost exclusively on fatty acids (this conserves ketone bodies for the brain's use).

However, skeletal muscle does not just consume fuels. It also provides substrates for the synthesis of fuels during the fasting state. During the first few days of fasting, there is tremendous muscle protein breakdown to provide glucogenic amino acids that are used by the liver to synthesize glucose. But, if the fasting continues for more than 3 weeks, the amount of protein degradation in skeletal muscle significantly slows, thereby decreasing the supply of glucogenic amino acids to the liver. The result is that serum glucose levels decrease further, secondary to decreased hepatic gluconeogenesis (due to decreased availability of glucogenic amino acids). The brain at this point now must rely almost exclusively on ketone bodies as a fuel source (and, conveniently, at about the same time, skeletal muscle stops using ketone bodies as a fuel source, so the two tissues do not compete).

During the first few days of fasting, glycogenolysis and gluconeogenesis occur with enough efficiency that the brain continues to rely exclusively on glucose as a fuel source. (Note that all hepatic glycogen stores are generally depleted within the 1st 10-18 hours of the fast, leaving only gluconeogenesis as a source for glucose). After the first few days of fasting, the brain starts to use ketone bodies synthesized by the liver, too. By about the 3rd week of a fast, the brain uses almost exclusively ketone bodies as a fuel source – simply because of less availability of glucose.

There are several eukaryotic DNA polymerases. The more important ones are as follows:

Pol alpha – acts as the primase

Pol beta – repairs DNA

Pol delta– repairs DNA and catalyzes DNA synthesis for elongation of the lagging strand

Pol epsilon – repairs DNA and catalyzes the DNA synthesis for elongation of the leading strand

Pol gamma – replicates, proofreads, and repairs DNA

Eukaryotic DNA is highly organized. The DNA is wrapped twice around a group of histones (8 histones total: (2) H2A, (2) H2B, (2) H3, and (2) H4). Such an arrangement is bead-like and is termed a nucleosome. Each nucleosome is connected to another nucleosome via "linker DNA." One histone, termed H1, is bound to each stretch of linker DNA. The resulting structure looks like a beaded necklace. The nucleosomes are then packed and wound closely together to form a structure known as a polynucleosome (a nucleofilament). The polynucleosome is coiled and "anchored" by scaffold protein. This then is organized to form a chromosome, distinct organized linear DNA arranged in the aforementioned manner.

There are 23 pairs of chromosomes in the human.

There are 3 major types of RNA:

1) transfer RNA (tRNA) – transfers amino acids to the ribosome
2) messenger RNA (mRNA) – is created from transcription of DNA and is used by the tRNA (and ribosome) to determine the sequence of amino acids needed for protein synthesis (translation).
3) ribosomal RNA (rRNA) – functions in the ribosome

A variety of mutations are associated with translation (the process of protein synthesis, guided by the code provided by mRNA). The code provided by the mRNA is classified according to codons, 3-nucleotide groups that "code" for a specific amino acid.

741

A silent mutation is one in which a mutated or changed codon is presented, but it still codes for the same amino acid as what should be placed in that location in that polypeptide chain.

A missense mutation is one in which the mRNA codon is altered in a manner that results in coding for an incorrect amino acid.

A nonsense mutation is one in which the altered codon is a termination codon, coding for premature termination of polypeptide synthesis.

Protein synthesis is comprised of 3 steps: 1) Initiation, 2) Elongation, and 3) Termination.

In initiation, mRNA binds to the small ribosome subunit. Initiation factors play a vital role in this process. The 5'-cap of the mRNA in eukaryotes is used to correctly position the mRNA on the ribosome. In prokaryotes, the Shine-Dalgarno sequence (a purine rich area of the mRNA) serves the same purpose, allowing the mRNA to bind to the 16S rRNA of the ribosome. In addition, during initiation, amino acids and tRNA join the complex. Amino acids are brought to the mRNA-ribosome complex via tRNA. mRNA codons are "recognized" by tRNA by virtue of tRNA's anti-codon binding to the mRNA's codon. The only way that binding can occur between the anti-codon and the codon is if their nucleotide sequences are complementary to one another (and the binding occurs in anti-parallel fashion). For instance, if the mRNA codon is UUG, then the tRNA anticodon must be AAU.

In elongation, the polypeptide chain is synthesized. It is created by the formation of peptide bonds between amino acids. All amino acids are added to the carboxyl end of the growing polypeptide chain. Elongation factors play a vital role in this process. The formation of the actual peptide bond between amino acids presented to the complex is catalyzed by peptidyl transferase, an enzyme that is actually not protein but, rather, made of 23S rRNA. After the peptide bond is formed, the ribosome moves to the next codon on the mRNA (this is called translocation), in preparation for placement of the next amino acid (remember, the mRNA codon determines what amino acid is added). Many ribosomes can translate an mRNA at a time, allowing for more rapid translation. The structure, all together with the many ribosomes attached, is termed a polysome.

In termination, the mRNA presents a termination codon (UAG, UAA, or UGA). Release factors are vital to the recognition of the termination codons. When recognized, the polypeptide that has been synthesized is released from the ribosome and the ribosome dissociates from the mRNA.

Biotechnology has allowed for vast changes in our understanding, evaluation, and manipulation of DNA.

Restriction enzymes, also known as restriction endonucleases, have been critical to this process. They are bacterial enzymes that are used in the laboratory setting to cleave double-stranded DNA at specific nucleotide sequences. The specific nucleotide sequences are known as restriction sites. The products of restriction enzyme action on DNA are termed restriction fragments, and represent fragments of DNA with well defined ends.

To clone a segment of DNA, DNA is typically cleaved by restriction enzymes. Then the fragments are individually joined to a larger DNA molecule known as the cloning vector (DNA vector molecule). A common cloning vector is the bacterial plasmid. The combination of the cloning vector with the restriction fragment is known as a recombinant DNA molecule. That recombinant DNA molecule is then introduced to organisms, such as bacteria, in which it and the organism replicate. This process is known as amplification (or getting more copies of the DNA). Once amplification has been completed, that DNA can be said to have been cloned. The cloned DNA is then purified from the organism and worked with as desired.

An alternative to DNA cloning is PCR, polymerase chain reaction. This method does not rely on the use of microorganisms for amplification of DNA fragments. As a result, it is very fast, enabling the lab to generate many copies of DNA in a few hours. DNA is denatured into 2 single-strands and then, using primers, is copied via DNA polymerase to create 2 double-strands of DNA. Then, those double strands are denatured (with heat) into 4 single-strands. DNA polymerase is used to copy those, yielding 4 double-strands. And, this process is continued repeatedly until enough copies are synthesized as desired. Because of its speed and sensitivity, PCR is used for forensic analysis of DNA evidence and for prenatal diagnosis of diseases such as cystic fibrosis.

Forensic DNA samples are usually so minute in quantity that amplification is necessary before they can be analyzed. That is why PCR is so helpful.

In a variety of clinical and basic sciences applications, one must identify what DNA fragment is present. The DNA fragments can be cloned or amplified, or simply obtained via restriction of a stretch of DNA of interest, and electrophoresed. There are multiple means by which to accomplish identification of the DNA fragment. One is by the use of probes. Probes are DNA fragments of known sequence that are tagged, frequently with a radioisotope. If the target DNA (DNA complementary to the probe) is present, the probe binds to it and its tag is used to locate the target DNA.

743

Probes can be used to not only identify target DNA, they can also be used to identify target mRNA. And, non-DNA probes, such as tagged antibodies, can be used to identify target proteins.

DNA of interest, whether cloned, amplified, or directly cleaved, can be electrophoresed (driven across a matrix such as agarose by electrical current). Then the DNA is denatured to single strands and transferred to nitrocellulose paper (simply by placing the paper onto the agarose gel). The probe is added to the paper and the process known as "hybridization" occurs (the probe binds to complementary DNA segments). Then, X-ray film is exposed to the hybridized specimen on the paper. Anything with bound probe will show up as black on the X-ray film. This technique is called Southern blotting.

A similar process is available to analysis of RNA. That process is termed Northern blotting.

Likewise, a somewhat similar process is available for the identification of proteins using antibody probes. That technique is termed Western blotting.

Southern = DNA
inbreed,

North = RNA
West = protein

Clinically, polymorphisms are very helpful clinically. They are minor variations in DNA that have no effect on the individual (vs. mutations that do have an effect). Polymorphisms can be studied by creating restriction fragment length polymorphisms (RFLPs). These RFLPs are created by subjecting the DNA in question (e.g., the DNA from a patient) to particular restriction enzymes. Then, the products are electrophoresed (different sized fragments move at different speeds through the gel, creating a unique pattern specific for each individual). The use and study of RFLPs is clinically useful for determining parentage of a child and for prenatal diagnosis of key diseases, such as PKU and sickle cell disease.

■■■

Gene therapy, also known as gene replacement therapy, is therapy in which cloned, normal DNA is inserted into the somatic cells (non-germ cells) of individuals with a defective gene that is causing a disease. A disease that has been successfully treated in this manner is severe combined immunodeficiency disease (SCIDs).

ELISA (pronounced "ee"-"lie"-"za") is enzyme-linked immunosorbent assay. It is used to detect the presence of particular proteins (and other molecules of interest). The probe is an antibody tagged with often some substance that will cause a change in color if antibody binding occurs. The amount or intensity of color produced can also, frequently, be used to quantitate the amount of the substance or protein of interest that is present. So, ELISAs are used qualitatively but also, frequently, quantitatively. ELISA assays are used for HIV screening. If positive, confirmatory testing is done with Western blotting. There are many more applications for ELISA in medicine and many other fields of science.

Appendix B

<u>Female Reproductive
System Disorders: Addendum</u>

Mayer-Rokitansky-Kuster-Hauser (MRKH) Syndrome
> Vaginal and/or uterine agenesis or dysgenesis
> Due to Mullerian agenesis or dysgenesis

Testicular Feminization Syndrome
> 46 XY, but have nonfunctional testosterone receptors
> <u>Findings</u>: have the beginning of a vagina with undescended testes (NO ovaries); phenotypically, externally appear as a female

Uterine Leiomyoma
> fibroid; uterine myoma
> Proliferation (benign) of uterine smooth muscle; hormonally responsive to estrogen (grow quicker during pregnancy or exposure to exogenous estrogen)
> Regress during menopause
> <u>Risk Factors</u>: US blacks
> <u>Signs/Symptoms</u>: menorrhagia, dysmenorrhea, dyspareunia, infertility, pelvic pain/pressure, +/- infertility, +/- urinary incontinence or constipation
> <u>Findings</u>: masses on or within muscular uterus, sometimes palpable as very firm, localized masses
> <u>Treatment</u>: progesterone, danazol, GnRH agonists — Leuprolide
> *steroid antagon that causes ⊖ feedback on pituitary*

Menopause
> cessation of menses, peak 52-53 y.o.
> <u>Signs/Symptoms</u>: hot flashes, amenorrhea, atrophic and dry vaginal mucosa
> May result in hirsutism and osteoporosis
> Elevated FSH and LH ↓estrogen

Hypogonadotropic hypogonadism

lack of hypothalamus or pituitary function results in inadequate gonadal function

Etiologies: pituitary pathology; Kallman's syndrome; tumors, TB, or sarcoid of hypothalamus, pituitary, or surrounding area; anorexia nervosa; exceedingly high stress; professional athletes; weight loss

Hypergonadotropic hypogonadism

lack of gonadal (ovarian) response to gonadotropins results in over activity of the pituitary and hypothalamus (hypergonadotropism) with no gonadal response (hypogonadism)

Asherman's Syndrome

intrauterine synechiae and adhesions

Often results in amenorrhea

Etiology: uterine surgery, infection, D&C (dilation and curettage), medical abortion

Adenomyosis

growth of endometrial glands and stroma into uterine musculature

Unknown etiology

Starts in 30's-40's, in parous women

Signs/Symptoms: dysmenorrhea, menorrhagia

Findings: diffusely large uterus that is soft

Dx: MRI

Treatment: analgesics, then hysterectomy

Endometriosis   endometrial tissue outside the endometrial
cavity
Likely due to retrograde menstruation out
the fallopian tubes into the peritoneal
cavity
Usually begins in 20's
Sometimes develop endometriomas
(cystic collection of endometriosis on the
ovary which, if filled with thick, dark, old
blood, is termed a chocolate cyst)
Risk Factors: black persons have the
LOWEST risk; (+) genetic predisposition
is a risk factor
Signs/Symptoms: dysmenorrhea,
dyspareunia, infertility, cyclic pelvic pain
Diagnosis: Requires DIRECT
visualization
Treatment: progesterone or danazol or
GnRH agonists

Ovarian Cysts   Two Types: functional cysts & neoplastic
growth

FUNCTIONAL CYSTS:

1.   Corpus Lutein Cyst
                    *formed after
                    ovulation
                    from the corpus
                    luteum
                    *enlarged or
                    hemorrhagic
                    corpus luteum that
                    fails to
                    resolve within 14 days
                    *causes a delay in
                    menstruation
                    *dull pelvic pain
                    *unilateral

2.   Follicular Cyst   *most common
*due to failure of
follicle to
rupture
*unilateral &
asymptomatic
*disappear within 60
days

3.   Theca Lutein Cyst

*filled with serous
fluid within cysts of
theca cells
*due to high, high,
high beta-hCG
stimulation from molar
pregnancy,
choriocarcinoma, or
clomiphene therapy
*B/L cysts
*pelvic discomfort &
high androgens
→hirsutism

B-hCG stimulate, Theca cells → androgens

NEOPLASTIC CYSTS

3. serous cystadenocarcinoma/cystadenoma
4. mucinous cystadenocarcinoma/cystadenoma

Uterine anatomic abnormalities
disorder of fusion of paramesonephric
(Mullerian) ducts
bicornuate uterus, bicornuate uterus with double
cervix, uterus didelphys with septate vagina

Savage's Syndrome   ovarian receptor defect
A type of ovarian failure, therefore →
amenorrhea (primary)

749

Turner's Syndrome   ovarian atresia, therefore ovarian failure
resulting in amenorrhea

AMENORRHEA

Potential sources of problems:

Primary amenorrhea		**Secondary amenorrhea**
Hypogonadotropic hypogonadism (e.g., Kallman's, Anatomic pathology such as tumors)	**HYPOTHALAMUS**	Hypogonadotropic hypogonadism (e.g., from anorexia nervosa, athletes, stress)
Hypogonadotropic hypogonadism (e.g. from anatomic pathology such as tumors, irradiation, hemosiderosis)	**ANT. PITUITARY**	Hypogonadotropic hypogonadism (e.g., TB, sarcoid, or hyperprolactinemia secondary to hi TSH, dopamine blockers pregnancy, breastfeeding, or tumor)
Hypergonadotropic hypogonadism (such as ovarian failure due Savage's or Turner's Syndrome) → lo estradiol with hi LH, FSH	**OVARY**	1) Hypergonadotropic hypogonadism (e.g. such as PREMATURE ovarian failure due to infection, early menopause) 2) PCOS
	UTERUS (Endometrium)	Asherman's Syndrome
Outflow tract disorders (e.g., imperforate hymen (marked by hematocolpos and cyclic pain) or Mayer Rokitansky Kuster Hauser Syndrome (with complete vaginal or uterine agenesis)	**VAGINA**	
Testicular Feminization	**OTHER**	

Appendix C

<u>Non-Malignant Testicular Disorders</u>
<u>(and related topics):Addendum</u>

TORSION   Twisting of testicle on its spermatic cord, impeding testicular blood supply
Sudden, Excruciating Testicular Pain!!! +/- abd pain with nausea and vomiting
<u>Predisposition</u>: developmental abnormality predisposes patient to torsion
<u>Etiology</u>: strenuous physical activity
<u>Findings</u>: swollen, tender, ELEVATED testicle; increased pain with elevation of testicle (Prehn's Sign); no transillumination of mass; testicle lies transversely instead of vertically
<u>Treatment</u>: immediate manual manipulation followed by surgery; testicle must be detorsed within 4-6 hours!! (if testicle is infarcted, it must be removed)

STRADDLE INJURY   Occurs as a result of a sudden, forceful fall onto groin
Very intense, excruciating initial pain
<u>Findings</u>: Hematuria, scrotal swelling, and (*via urethrography*) extravasation of urine into scrotum
<u>Treatment</u>: surgery

APPENDIX TESTES TORSION   Severe pain
Findings: blue dot sign
Treatment: surgery

CRYPTORCHIDISM   Undescended testes
Spontaneous descent does not occur beyond 1 year old
Associated with increased risk of tumor, infertility, and torsion
Frequently associated with inguinal hernia
Risk Factors: prematurity
Findings: empty scrotum
Treatment: surgery at early age

CHYLOCELE   Accumulation of lymph fluid in tunica vaginalis
Etiology: elephantiasis (filariasis) due to Wuchereria bancrofti

SPERMATOCELE   Cystic accumulation of sperm in epididymis
Findings: cystic swelling in epididymis, very tender to palpation

HYDROCELE   Clear serous fluid accumulation within tunica vaginalis
Occurs secondary to testicular infections, tumors
Findings: scrotum enlarged, and feels smooth and resilient; translucent on transillumination

VARICOCELE   Dilated cluster of veins within the scrotum, just above the testicle
"Bag of worms" on palpation, which is worsened with standing; slow, gradual onset
Decreases fertility
Usually asymptomatic, but get a heavy, achy scrotal feeling (especially with running)
>98% occur on left
Right varicocele or acute onset left or right varicocele should prompt search for anything that increases venous system pressures (e.g., blockade secondary to abdominal tumors, etc.)
Findings: bumpy, "bag of worms" feel above testicle

HEMATOCELE   Blood accumulation within tunica vaginalis
Occurs secondary to trauma, torsion, or bleeding
disorders
Findings: tense, enlarged scrotum; does not
transilluminate

TESTICULAR MASSES   Neoplastic ones tend to be hard,
"marble-sized mass", nontender
Nonmalignant ones tend to not be as hard
(although they can be), but also are
usually nontender…etiologies: TB,
Tertiary syphilis (gummas)

TESTICULAR DYSGENESIS   Ambiguous external genitalia in
a chromosomal male
Mullerian structures absent
Findings: B/L inguinal swelling
with ambiguous male genitalia
Treatment: orchiectomy with
hormone replacement therapy

ORCHITIS   Inflammation of the testes
Findings: pain +/- swelling; if acute, scrotal skin
is also erythematous and scrotum is markedly
enlarged
Etiologies: mumps, syphilis, gonorrhea

ACUTE EPIDIDYMITIS

Inflammation of the epididymis
Usually of gradual onset
Findings: intense, unbearable, debilitating pain with surrounding swelling and erythema; fever, pyuria
Etiologies: largely age dependent…..

BOYS: secondary to congenital genitourinary tract abnormalities
MEN <35 y.o.: Neisseria, Chlamydia
MEN ≥ 35 y.o.: secondary to acquired anatomic abnormalities
ANY AGE: traumatic causes or "chemical acute epididymitis"

B/L MICROORCHIDISM

Small testes
Etiologies: Klinefelter's, Myotonic Dystrophy, Secondary hypogonadism

U/L MICROORCHIDISM

One small testicle
Etiologies: atrophy secondary to mumps, syphilis, trauma

B/L MACROORCHIDISM

Large testes
Etiology: Fragile X Syndrome

Appendix D
Rapid Review of OMM Principles

- Acute somatic dysfunction presents with the same features as acute inflammation.

- Chronic somatic dysfunction presents with the same features as chronic inflammation.

- The restrictive barrier is also known as the pathologic barrier.

- The restrictive barrier represents a barrier to having normal, free movement, most specifically a barrier to reaching one's physiologic barrier.

- A restrictive barrier is, because it is a barrier, the opposite of "freedom."

- Although we name somatic dysfunction for its freedom, remember it is still somatic DYSFUNCTION.

- So, assuming there is already DYSFUNCTION, within that dysfunction, for diagnosis and nomenclature purposes, we find the "freedoms" that lie within that dysfunction.

- Dysfunction = Somatic dysfunction = Nomenclature = Diagnosis

- The dysfunction itself is due to a restriction, but that does not mean that other movements are restricted.

- Thus when naming a dysfunction, we find the "freedom." That is, in the example of rotation, the side to which we can we rotate the most (e.g., have the most freedom at rotating) DESPITE the restriction caused by the dysfunction.

- If there were no dysfunction, we would rotate evenly on both sides.

- If there is dysfunction, we rotate more to one side than the other; the side to which we rotate more is the side of freedom for rotation, and that is the rotational component we assign to the dysfunction. So, if the structure we are assessing is in dysfunction and rotates more to the right than the left, we say it is a rotated right dysfunction.

- The restrictive barrier or restriction is always on the opposite side; after all, restriction is the opposite of "freedom."

- Hence, if the structure we are assessing rotates more to the right, we know that the restriction is on the left.

- Sidebending is handled similarly, such that if we sidebend more to the right than the left, we have a sidebending right dysfunction with a left restriction.

- Thus, if something is rotated right, sidebent right, for example, we know that it is restricted in being able to rotate to the left and sidebend to the left. Thus, any asymmetric movement indicates that there is dysfunction. Thus, any time we move better in one direction than another, that means that there is restriction in the opposite direction.

- The position in the sagittal plane (flexion, neutral, sidebending) that is used to name the dysfunction is also named for ITS freedom – not for any freedom it gives to rotation or sidebending, but for the most freedom overall that can be exhibited while in a particular position in the sagittal plane.

- Thus, flexion, neutral, and extension for dysfunction nomenclature are determined by which of those positions affords the most freedom (least overall restriction) to the spine while in that particular position.

- The more rotated or sidebent we are to one side, by nature, the less freedom is also demonstrated in the sagittal plane position (flexion, extension, neutral) that promotes that dysfunction. We are, in essence, locked up into a dysfunctional position. We are demonstrating the positions that maximize restriction (if there is more freedom to one side, then that means that there is restriction on the other, e.g., dysfunction exists).

- Conversely, the more symmetric our rotational and sidebending abilities, the more likelihood we have for also having FREE and easy sagittal movement.

- Thus, if we are rotated right and sidebent left, and this is most pronounced in non-neutral positions (e.g., flexion and extension), that means that we are most in dysfunction and most "locked up" when flexed or extended. That is not freedom.

- Remember, we do NOT name the movements in the sagittal plane by what way rotation is more free or what way sidebending is more free – after all, we already did that when we named the rotational and sidebending components.

- Instead, if we are rotated right and sidebent left, and this is most pronounced in non-neutral positions, that means that we will have more symmetric movement (to right AND left, in terms of rotation and sidebending) whenever we are neutral. That means that we are then more free to undergo a sagittal movement – but that freedom is best in neutral, a position in which we are least locked up and MOST FREE.

- Hence, if we are most free (e.g., experience less dysfunction) in neutral, then, because we name the dysfunctions for their freedoms, the dysfunction in this case would be neutral.

- For instance, if a patient is rotated left and this rotational finding is most noticeable in neutral and least noticeable in flexion, this would be a FR_L somatic dysfunction.

- Fryette mechanics ONLY applies to the thoracic and lumbar spine. It states that, a neutral dysfunction (Type I dysfunction) features sidebending and rotation to the opposite side. It also states that a non-neutral dysfunction (Type II dysfunction; flexion or extension) features sidebending and rotation to the same side.

  Flexion and extension move to the same side:

  Neutral moves to the opposite side:

- Fryette mechanics do NOT apply to the cervical spine or the sacrum. The sacrum does not have individual vertebral segments, as they are all fused. And, the cervical spine follows the cervical motion rules.

- In the thoracic spine or lumbar spine, if there were a FR_L dysfunction, we know that the sidebending component for the nomenclature and diagnosis would be S_L. We know this because Fryette mechanics state that flexion dysfunctions feature sidebending and rotation to the same side.

- If there were a NS_R dysfunction of the thoracic or lumbar spine, that would mean that it would have to be rotated left to yield NS_RR_L; that follows Fryette mechanics.

- Cervical motion rules dictate how the cervical segments move. C0 (occiput; OA) and C1 (atlas; AA) always, REGARDLESS of the sagittal positioning of freedom, will have rotation and sidebending to the opposite side.

- Therefore, if C0 is ER_R, it would have to be sidebent left. The rotational and sidebending relationships in the cervical spine are not dictated by the sagittal position, as they are in the thoracic and lumbar spine. Instead, the rotational and sidebending relationship is determined solely by what cervical vertebral segment is in dysfunction.

- C2-C7 always, REGARDLESS of the freedom of position sagittally, will have rotation and sidebending to the same side.

- Thus, $C4NR_R$ will have S_R because it is C4 that determines the rotation-sidebending relationship.

- Forward sacral torsions always have the axis and rotation on the same side; think

- So, if the sacrum is rotated right on a right axis, it has to be a forward sacral torsion.

- With a backward sacral torsion, the axis and rotation are opposite to one another:

- So, if the sacrum is rotated left on a right axis, it has to be a backward sacral torsion.

- If there is a torsion, <u>the axis will always be on the opposite side of the most evident pathology at the sacral superior sulcus</u>. If the right sacral superior sulcus is determined to be deep, the left ILA will be shallow *if this is a torsion*. After all, torsion means to torse or twist around, so while one side is up, the opposite side (both laterally and longitudinally opposite) will be down. Since the SUPERIOR SACRAL SULCUS is deep, that means the sacrum is dipping forward. And, we already determined that this is a torsion because of the particular type of ILA involvement. So, this must be a forward sacral torsion. With that being said, remember that the most evident pathology at the superior sacral sulcus was on the right. That means that, for a torsion, the axis must be on the left, the side opposite of the pathology. Hence we know this is a forward sacral torsion ("forward" because the superior sacral sulcus is dipping forward, and a torsion because the ILA and sulcus together are demonstrating torsion-like movements) and we know that we must have a left axis (because of the right superior sulcus findings demonstrating that the pathology is on the right), so that means that we must also be rotated left (because a forward sacral torsion always is featured by an ipsilateral axis and rotation). So, to produce these findings, the sacrum would have to be rotated left on a left axis – a forward sacral torsion.

- Anytime there is disease, damage, injury, illness, or dysfunction of a body part, organ, region, or tissue, the body's protective mechanisms are activated.

- The protective mechanisms include the fight or flight response.

- The fight or flight response is mediated by the sympathetic nervous system.

- Thus, any disease, damage, injury, illness, or dysfunction of a body part, organ, region, or tissue results in activation of sympathetic nerve fibers that serve that particular part, organ, region, or tissue.

- The activation causes afferent signals to be delivered to the spinal cord. The afferent signals go to specific segments of the spinal cord, specifically those segments that provide sympathetic innervation to that particular part, organ, region, or tissue. For instance, the T5 region of the spinal cord serves, sympathetically, the liver. Thus, in this latter instance, if there were pathology at the liver (e.g., hepatitis B), the T5 spinal cord segment would receive afferent impulses via autonomic fibers.

- Excessive volume or chronic delivery of impulses to the cord causes the spinal cord to become facilitated; such facilitation means that there is now a lower threshold to activation, allowing for easy and ready impulses to be delivered FROM that spinal cord segment to any part of the body served by that spinal cord segment. The outgoing impulses can be in the form of sympathetic innervation, to produce a sympathetic response, in another tissue. The outgoing impulses can also cause skeletal muscle activation to produce hypertonicity and spasms. Referred pain can also be produced.

- When a pathology causes spinal cord facilitation that ultimately causes a reflex stimulation elsewhere due to the facilitation, that is termed a reflex arc.

- Thus, for example, chronic hepatitis B would cause chronic afferent stimulation of the T5 spinal cord segment. With time or with increasing severity, the T5 region of the spinal cord can become facilitated. Once that happens, outgoing impulses to those regions served by T5 can be affected. For instance, outgoing sympathetic impulses via T5 can affect the stomach, since the stomach is also sympathetically supplied by T5. Sympathetic stimulation of the stomach causes decreased stomach function and decreased gastric emptying along with decreased digestive actions. The result is nausea, a common complaint by those with chronic hepatitis B.

- Referred pain is a common manifestation of facilitation with a reflex arc.

- Sympathetic responses, like those that can be PRODUCED via facilitation, will be always geared for immediate survival; so, depending on the regions affected, the inciting pathology, and the level of the spinal cord that is facilitated, some sympathetic responses can include ileus or constipation, tachycardia, increased gluconeogenesis, decreased glomerular filtration rate, uterine relaxation, urinary and fecal retention, and decreased biliary flow; in other words, immediate survival mechanisms (like increased heart rate, provision of glucose to the blood stream) will prevail while those mechanisms not needed for immediate survival (though needed for long term survival), such as peristalsis, urination and defecation, and labor (during pregnancy) will be inhibited.

- Sympathetic responses can also be generated systemically directly by the adrenal medulla's release of epinephrine and norepinephrine into the bloodstream, an action that occurs secondary to an extremely dangerous or life-threatening event.

Appendix E

<u>Medico-Legal Basics</u>

Criminal liability = accountability for a crime, such as a felony. Felonies include failing to report suspected child abuse or elder abuse, child abuse, euthanasia, unlawful distribution of controlled substances, and death of a patient due to gross misconduct. Criminal violations are pursued by the state or federal government and are punishable by fines or imprisonment.

Civil liability = accountability for a civil offense, such as breach of contract, medical malpractice, invasion of privacy, invasion of person, and defamation. Civil offenses are pursued by the victim or representatives of the victim, and result in monetary awards to the victim.

> **Breach of Contract** = failure to comply with the terms of a valid contract, namely the "contract" that exists within a doctor-patient relationship. There two main types of breach of contract in medicine are abandonment and breach of confidentiality.

> > **Abandonment** = failure to continue to provide medical care without following very specific rules (cannot sever doctor-patient relationship unless serious legally acceptable issues exist) AND giving ample notice to patient well in advance of cessation of service (exception: failure to provide services due to the doctor's death allows for notification after the death, but it must be immediate to all patients)

Breach of Confidentiality = failure to keep patient records and information confidential; breach can occur via oral, written, or visual communication, even to a passerby who is not actually "in" the conversation.

Medical Malpractice = Medical Negligence. Is a type of civil liability. In order to be a medical malpractice, it must meet the "4 D's of Negligence" rule:
1. Duty (e.g., there was a doctor-patient relationship)
2. Dereliction (the physician did not follow the standard of care, either by doing something or omitting something that is part of that standard)
3. Damages (injury or measurable damages occurred)
4. Direct Cause (the damages were a DIRECT result of the actions or inactions of the physician)

Res Ipsa Loquitur = "the thing speaks for itself." Represents medical malpractice in which duty and dereliction are obvious and unquestionable. All that has to be proven is that damages occurred, and that they were a direct result of the dereliction.

Boards Boot Camp High-Yield Compendium

Invasion of Person or Privacy = Battery (invasion of person) or unauthorized publicity (verbal, visual, written) of a patient's information, body, exam, or conversation.

Informed Consent = Act by which a person voluntarily gives permission for a medical professional to do something specific, after having been informed of the risks, the benefits, and alternate options, and risks of not doing anything at all; in medicine, that refers to consent for medical examination, evaluation, management, treatment, and procedures.

Battery = in the medical field, means intentional examining, touching, treating, or performing any procedure on a patient without their consent. Is a type of civil liability, classified as invasion of person.

Assault = intentionally physically harming another person

Defamation = either **Libel** (written) or **Slander** (spoken), and is the dissemination, in any form, of damaging, false information about another person or entity (which must be heard/read/seen by a person or entity other than the person or entity about which this information exists). For instance, saying something false and damaging to a fellow physician IN PRIVATE with only you and that physician present is not defamation, although it is unprofessional and unethical. Generally, can result in one medical group suing another, etc. Is a type of civil liability.

Respondeat superior = means "let the master speak," and is translated to mean that the physician is legally responsible for any acts or inactions by their employees that result in any form of patient harm.

Primum non nocer = above all, do no harm; this means that the benefits of any patient care must outweigh the risks.

Capacity = medical competence = capacity to make medical decisions for oneself

Incapacity = one's inability to make medical decisions for themselves for THAT specific period of time for a SPECIFIC medical action or inaction. Only physicians can determine capacity; the most legally defensible determinations are made by psychiatrists since they enlist the legal requirements to assess all medical parameters, the medical condition, the seriousness and acuity of the situation, the mental state of the patient, the patient's personal belief system and goals, and relate that into a determination as to whether a patient is able to make a decision for themselves that is consistent with what their typical health preferences would be. Incapacity is not global or permanent and is supposed to be limited to a particular medical action or inaction for a specific limited period of time (wherein the patient is re-evaluated for capacity).

Involuntary treatment requires that the patient be mentally ill AND be a danger to self or others. Alternatively, for instance, being a danger to others, but not mentally ill, is a criminal issue, not a medical issue.

Treatment of pediatric patients requires parental or custodial consent UNLESS the case is or involves:
1) Emergency
2) Pregnancy (exception in some states is abortion) 20 weeks
3) Treatment of STDs (with some states applying some limitations)
4) Child is designated by a judge to be a mature minor, or child is emancipated (some limitations to the latter may apply)

Advanced Directives = directives to be followed in the event that the patient is incapacitated.

Living will = written instructions regarding health care that are to be followed in the event that the patient becomes incapacitated

Power of Attorney = a person who is designated by the patient, during a time of capacity, to act as a surrogate for health care decision-making on behalf of the patient should the patient become incapacitated

DNR = Do Not Resuscitate = CPR is withheld (but other treatment is NOT!). Is a written decree by the patient, obtained through informed consent by the physician.

Boards Boot Camp High-Yield Compendium

Medicare = healthcare funding for the elderly (> 65 years of age) or the disabled (is part of Social Security)

A hospital
B office
C plus
D drugs

Medicaid = healthcare funding for the poor (e.g., those on Welfare)

CHIP = Children's Health Insurance Program = government-funded health insurance for all uninsured children, regardless of family income level

Managed Care Organizations = health insurance models, and include PPOs and HMOs

HMO = Health Maintenance Organization. The physician, group, or hospital is an employee of the insurance company, and receives a set amount of money each month based on the number of patients "assigned" to them (regardless of how many patients have been seen, treated, etc). Any visits to specialists require a referral.

PPO = Preferred Provider Organization = Participating Provider Organization = physician, group or hospital is under contractual agreement with the insurance company to provide healthcare at a significantly reduced rate to the insurance company's members. Visits to specialists do not require a referral. However, if the patient goes to a specialist or other physician who is "out-of-network" (code word for not being under contractual agreement with the insurance company), only a certain percentage of what the insurance company deems itself as an "allowable" cost for that service will be covered.

Fee-for-service is the model of practicing medicine while not accepting insurance; the patient pays the physician upfront. Patients frequently then submit claims themselves, if they do have insurance and if it is a covered service. This model is common among aesthetic dermatologists and plastic surgeons.

Boutique medicine is a type of fee-for-service practice. However, instead of paying per visit or service, the patient pays, typically, an annual fee; that usually allows the patient unlimited visits with the physician, and often many other included ancillary services, as well. Usually, such practices rely heavily on preventive medicine and wellness visits, in order to avoid the time and cost of the many visits needed should a disease arise.

Patient Protection and Affordable Care Act – commonly called Obamacare (or federal health care law). A US federal statute designed to decrease the number of uninsured individuals, to allow those with pre-existing conditions to be insured, and to reduce current healthcare costs (current estimates are that upwards of 60% of healthcare costs are incurred for under- or uninsured individuals, and those costs are paid for by the remaining 40% who are insured and by government entities).

Appendix F   BIOSTATISTICS

This topic plays a relatively small role for COMLEX, but a much more significant role for USMLE.

Sensitivity = something that is very sensitive to anomalies

Sensitive tests are preferred for screening tests since they can identify anomalies that exist; unless they are specific, too, they will not be able to, however, identify what the cause of the anomaly is

SENSITIVITY =   (Number of positive test results among those who have the disease)/(Total number of people with the disease)

Specificity = something that can specify exactly what the disease is (its results are specific)

Specific tests are preferred for confirmatory tests since they can specify what exactly the disease is.

SPECIFICITY =   (Number of negative test results among those without the disease)/(Total number of people without the disease)

False Positive Ratio = the ratio of test results that were positive despite the person being free of the disease

FALSE POSITIVE RATIO = 1 – specificity

Prevalence = the total number of people in a population who have the Disease

A disease that has high prevalence is one that is occurring in a lot of people in the population; an example would be upper respiratory infections in winter time in temperate climates.

Incidence = the number of NEW cases of a disease within a population with a given period of time

Think of incidence as incidents – how many incidents (e.g., new cases) have there been in that population in that period of time? A disease has a high incidence if there have been a lot of new cases in a certain period of time; for instance, if there is a "break out" of measles in January in Southern California, it could be said that there was a high incidence of measles in Southern California in January. However, if it only affected 20 people, when compared to the population of Southern California, it could be said that measles has a low prevalence in that region (based on this case).

Prevalence > Incidence indicates chronic disease
Prevalence = Incidence indicates acute disease

Mortality = the number of people who DIE from the disease in a given period of time

Positive Predictive Value (PPV) = the probability of a patient having the disease if their test result is positive

This really determines the accuracy of the test; if the positive predictive value is low, it means that patients who have positive test results have a high likelihood of NOT having the disease. In other words, a low positive predictive value would mean that the test is not an accurate tool for ruling out a diagnosis

Additionally, unlike specificity or sensitivity, PPV values are also influenced by the prevalence of the disease. PPV will always be higher in populations for whom the disease has a high prevalence (simply because the number of the people with the disease is so high – try it out with the equation below).

PPV = (Number of people with the disease who had a positive test result)/(Number of people who had a positive test result)

Negative Predictive Value (NPV) = the probability of a patient NOT having the disease if their test result is negative

This determines how much one can accurately rely on a negative test result as really being able to rule in a disease. If the negative predictive value is low, that means that the test is not very accurate and that there is still a good chance that the patient has the disease, despite a negative test result. Additionally, unlike specificity or sensitivity, NPV values are also influenced by the prevalence of the disease. NPV will always be lower in populations for whom the disease has a high prevalence (simply because the number of healthy people will be so low – try it out with the equation below).

NPV = (Number of healthy people with negative test results)/(Total number of people who have a negative test result)

Odds Ratio = Estimates the risk for anyone in the population of getting the disease

This is only able to be used if the prevalence is not excessive. It is frequently used in case-control studies of disease. If the odds ratio is high, it means that anyone has a high chance of getting the disease.

Odds Ratio = [(Number of people who were exposed who got the disease) x (Number of people who were NOT exposed who did NOT get the disease)]/[(Number of people who were exposed to the disease but did not get the disease)x(Number of people who were not known to be exposed to the disease but DID get the disease)]

Relative Risk = Determines a ratio that compares the risk for those who were exposed of actually getting the disease as compared to the risk for those who were NOT exposed of getting the disease

Basically, it allows one to determine what risk the exposure itself presents; in other words, if a patient is exposed to the disease, what is the risk they will get the disease? (as opposed to odds ratio which answers the question: What is the chance of a patient getting the disease?).

Relative Risk = [(Number of people who were exposed who also have the disease/(Number of people who were exposed who also have the disease + Number of people who were exposed who do NOT have the disease)]/[(Number of people who were NOT exposed who DO have the disease)/(Number of people who were NOT exposed who DO have the disease + Number of people who were NOT exposed who DO NOT have the disease)]

Standard deviation - uses a normal Gaussian distribution ("bell curve") to determine where results fall as compared to others in the population. +/- one standard deviation includes 68% of the population tested. +/- two standard deviations includes 95% of the population being tested. And, +/- three standard deviations includes almost all (99.7%) of the population.

Terms to Know:

Reliability = the dependability of a test; it is determined by how reproducible the test results are.

Validity = a determination of how appropriate the test is for a given situation; in other words, does it test what it is supposed to test.

Precision = consistency of a test (the test may not be accurate, but if it consistently gives the same result, regardless of whether it is right or wrong, it is precise)

Accuracy = Trueness of test result; it truly reflects the condition being tested

Mean = average

Median = ½ of the population is below the median, and ½ is above the median

Null Hypothesis (H$_0$) = the statement that there is NO correlation or association between a disease and certain risk factors (or other parameters under study). If the results of a study support the null hypothesis, it means that no association was found between the risk factors and the disease

Type I Error (α) = A type of error that arises from a study in which the study states that there was an effect (due to the drug, risk factor, etc) when, in fact, there was NO effect. Due to this error, the null hypothesis is rejected (although it should not be – which is why this is called an error).

p = the probability of making a type I error; for instance, if the p < 0.10, then there is less than a 10% chance that the data will indicate that there was an effect that really was NOT there. Obviously, studies need low p values.

Type II Error (β) = A type of error that arises from a study in which the study states that there was NOT an effect (due to the drug, risk factor, etc) when, in fact, there was an effect. Due to this error, the null hypothesis is supported (although it should not have been – which is why this is called an error)

β = the probability of making a type II error

TYPES OF STUDIES and ANALYSES:

Clinical Trial = a study done as an experiment to assess the therapeutic benefit of certain treatments. Is the standard method prior to getting FDA approval and release of a drug to the market.

Cohort Study = a study done usually in real-time (e.g., current patients are used in the study); used to follow disease development and progression between populations with and without certain risk factors. Is also known as an Observational Cohort. Goal: Study the EFFECT OF risk factors and better characterize those risk factors

Case-Control Study = Used to follow patients already known to have and not have a disease (2 different populations), wherein the two populations are studied to identify risk factors for those diseases. Goal: Study those with a disease and, by comparing them with people who do not have the disease, identify WHAT the risk factors are

Boards Boot Camp High-Yield Compendium

Cross-Sectional Survey = a study done to determine correlations and associations between variables, and includes the study of <u>one</u> patient population in which multiple variables affecting their health are studied. <u>Correlation coefficients</u> are determined: +1 means there is perfect correlation between the variable and the disease (such as a living environment or social habit and the development of disease – for instance, smoking causes lung cancer); 0 means that there is no correlation (e.g., there is no correlation between smoking and the development of coxa valgum); -1 means that there is a negative correlation (e.g., smoking reduces that disease or some aspect of that disease – for instance, smoking reduces the number of flares in ulcerative colitis).

Meta-analysis = the collection of data from multiple studies to generate statistically more reliable data

Prospective Study = any study done here and now on current patients or subjects; cohort studies commonly are this type of study

Retrospective Study = any study in which medical records and data collected prior to the study are analyzed; case control studies are usually retrospective

Boards Boot Camp High-Yield Compendium

INDEX

Boards Boot Camp High-Yield Compendium

M

MAC, see *Mycobacterium avium complex*
Macrophage, 25-26, 28, 57, 65, 86, 115, 142, 177, 223, 227, 263, 369, 408, 570
Mad cow disease, 358
Major histocompatibility complex, 26, 28, 67, 267, 276, 361
Malpractice, 762
MCHC, 31-32
Measles, 163, 340, 345-348, 350, 357, 723, 769
Mebendazole, 719
Medicaid, 766
Medicare, 766
Medulla, 507, 523-525, 622, 625, 631, 639, 640-642, 646, 702-703
Melanin, 43, 165, 169, 417, 422
Mental retardation (see intellectual disability)
Mesoderm, 215, 253, 612-614, 652, 654
Metabolic acidosis, 554-556, 559, 571
MHC (see major histocompatibility complex)
Midbrain, 622, 626, 631-633, 646, 702
Milwaukee protocol, 355
Mitochondrial inheritance, 40, 42
Monocyte, 25, 29
mRNA, 28, 462-464, 466-467, 505, 741-742, 744
Muscle spindle, 512
Mycobacterium, 36, 68, 233, 259, 262, 271, 308-309, 313-314, 364-365
Mycobacterium avium complex, 68, 314, 364-365
Mycoplasma, 77, 119, 261-262, 272, 307, 725

N

NAD, 418, 449, 454, 458-460, 457, 732, 734
Narcissistic personality disorder, 599
Narcolepsy, 60
Necator americanus, 391
Neisseria, 141, 263, 271, 273, 281-283, 294, 754
Neonate, 114, 195, 252, 273, 278, 283, 288, 321-322, 332, 334, 518, 703
Neuraminidase, 343-344, 410, 723
Neurohypophysis, 657-658
Neurosyphilis, 221, 317, 606
Neurotransmitter, 43, 265, 293, 419, 478, 486-492, 495, 497, 500, 502-504, 599, 727
Nifurtimox, 378, 716
Nitric oxide, 25, 263, 496, 504, 574
NK cell, 25
Norepinephrine, 43, 232, 396, 417, 486-489, 492-494, 497, 528, 570, 572-573, 599, 654, 760

O

Obsessive-compulsive personality disorder, 600
Oculomotor nerve, 621, 627, 632
Oncogene, 37, 82, 163, 171, 337
Optic nerve, 614, 617-618, 623, 627, 629-630, 644, 701

P

p53, 37, 143, 152, 163, 171, 328-329
Paget's disease, 160, 204
Pancreatitis, 43, 61, 194, 243, 726
Panic disorder, 601
Paragonimus, 383-384, 386
Parotid gland, 113, 346, 499, 562
Patient Protection and Affordable Care Act, 767

PDGF (see platelet derived growth factor)
Pedigree, 40, 42
Pentamidine, 379
Peptic ulcer disease, 62, 246, 300, 705, 726
Peptidoglycan, 260-261, 320
Peroneal nerve, 685-686, 688-689
Peyer's patch, 296, 329, 667
Phenylalanine, 43, 298, 416-417, 422-423, 445, 453, 733, 737
Phenylketonuria, 43, 422
Placenta, 38, 149, 155, 245, 316-317, 324, 337, 361, 583, 612-613, 615
Plasmid, 743
Platelet-derived growth factor, 28
Plummer-Vinson syndrome, 79
Pneumococcus (see *Streptococcus pneumoniae*)
Pneumocystis, 67-68, 364-365, 375-376
Pneumonia, 208, 216, 263, 272-273, 278, 294, 298, 301, 304-308, 322-324, 329, 337, 343, 347-348, 357, 364-365, 370, 375
Pons, 489, 626, 631, 635-638, 646
Potassium, 125, 138, 231, 233, 470, 474, 481-482, 484, 488, 530-531, 544-545, 559, 565-566, 569, 598
Power of attorney, 765
PPO, 766
Prader-Willi syndrome, 59
Preterm delivery, 584
Primary biliary cirrhosis, 33-34, 181-182
Prolactin, 214, 228, 572, 659, 661, 750
Prostaglandin, 25, 396-397, 404, 409, 545, 563, 570, 582, 713, 715
Prostate, 38, 120, 170, 576, 592, 706, 709, 716
Pseudopolyp, 168, 174
PUD (see peptic ulcer disease)

Q

Q wave, 103, 532
Quadriceps, 684, 693

R

Rabies, 326, 340, 355-356
Radial nerve, 680-681, 691-692, 704
Raxibacumab, 286
Rectum, 120, 141, 168, 174, 278, 385, 498, 662, 707
Recurrent laryngeal nerve, 656, 673-675, 710-711
Reed-Sternberg cell, 83
Reiter's syndrome, 60, 296-297, 299, 302, 321
REM, 597-598
Res ipsa loquitur, 762
Respiratory acidosis, 555-556
Respondeat superior, 764
Rh factor, 36, 77
Rotator cuff, 678-680

S

Salmonella, 61, 273, 284, 294, 296, 321
Sensitivity, 768-770
Sepsis, 113, 173, 179, 278, 288
Shigella, 275, 284, 294, 297, 321
SLE (see systemic lupus erythematosus)
Sodium, 220, 231, 233, 470, 472, 474-476, 478-484, 487, 495, 504, 513, 530-531, 535, 542, 551, 546, 560-562, 565, 571-572, 639, 665-666, 716, 727-728
Specificity, 768-770
Spontaneous abortion, 584

Streptococcus, 36, 61, 105-108, 118, 123, 127, 129, 251, 263, 271-273, 278-281, 294, 728
Streptococcus agalactiae, 273, 278
Streptococcus bovis, 278
Streptococcus pneumoniae, 61, 107, 118, 263, 272-273, 278, 294, 728
Streptococcus pyogenes, 106, 108, 127, 251, 278-281, 728
Systemic lupus erythematosus, 33-34, 36, 60, 63, 77, 106, 126, 128, 224

T

Tenofovir, 721
Terrible triad, 686-687
Tetanus, 265, 287-288, 293, 520, 673
Thiamine (see vitamin B1)
TNF (see tumor necrosis factor)
Toxoplasmosis, 68, 362, 364-365, 376
Transforming growth factor, 29
Triceps, 646, 680-681, 693
Trifluridine, 720
Triglyceride, 194, 396-397, 400-402, 408, 445, 449, 452-453, 665-666, 733-734, 739
Trimethoprim, 139, 177, 315, 365, 376, 726, 728
Troponin, 103, 484, 514-515
Tumor necrosis factor, 25, 28-29, 263
Tumor suppressor gene, 37, 143, 152, 163, 169, 171, 212, 328, 339
Tyrosine, 416-417, 423, 445, 453, 500, 506, 733, 737

U

Umbilical artery, 615
Umbilical cord, 440, 615
Umbilical ligament, 615
Umbilical stump, 292
Umbilical vein, 615
Umbilicus, 615, 645, 649, 705

V

Vanillyl mandelic acid, 232
Varicella, 335
Vibrio, 284, 294, 298- 299
Vibrio cholerae, 298
Virchow's triad, 85
Visual field, 629-630, 710
Vitamin B1, 227, 446, 448, 544, 606
Vitamin B12, 32, 78, 80, 163, 175-176, 226, 254, 388, 449, 565, 606, 734
VMA (see vanillyl mandelic acid)

W

Waddling gait, 693
Wen, 694
Widowmaker, 652-653

X

X-linked, 40-42, 45-46, 55, 57, 70, 75, 224, 422
X-ray, 33, 110, 113, 118-119, 172, 174, 198, 256, 286, 309, 346, 744

Y

Yolk (egg), 406, 447
Yolk sac, 38, 145, 149, 611-612, 615
Yolk stalk, 615-616

Z

Zanamivir, 723, 343
Zollinger-Ellison syndrome, 246

Boards Boot Camp High-Yield Compendium

Boards Boot Camp High-Yield Compendium

781